T0270876

ROUTLEDGE LIBRARY EDITIONS: AGING

Volume 3

LIFE AFTER A DEATH

LIFE AFTER A DEATH

A Study of the
Elderly Widowed

ANN BOWLING
AND
ANN CARTWRIGHT

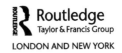

Routledge
Taylor & Francis Group

LONDON AND NEW YORK

First published in 1982 by Tavistock Publications Ltd

This edition first published in 2024
by Routledge
4 Park Square, Milton Park, Abingdon, Oxon OX14 4RN

and by Routledge
605 Third Avenue, New York, NY 10158

Routledge is an imprint of the Taylor & Francis Group, an informa business

British Library Cataloguing in Publication Data
A catalogue record for this book is available from the British Library

ISBN: 978-1-032-67433-9 (Set)
ISBN: 978-1-032-71500-1 (Volume 3) (hbk)
ISBN: 978-1-032-71607-7 (Volume 3) (pbk)
ISBN: 978-1-032-71606-0 (Volume 3) (ebk)

DOI: 10.4324/9781032716060

Publisher's Note
The publisher has gone to great lengths to ensure the quality of this reprint but points out that some imperfections in the original copies may be apparent.

Disclaimer
The publisher has made every effort to trace copyright holders and would welcome correspondence from those they have been unable to trace.

Ann Bowling
and Ann Cartwright

Institute for Social Studies
in Medical Care

Life After A Death

A Study of the
Elderly Widowed

TAVISTOCK PUBLICATIONS
LONDON AND NEW YORK

First published in 1982 by
Tavistock Publications Ltd
11 New Fetter Lane, London EC4P 4EE

Published in the USA by
Tavistock Publications
in association with Methuen, Inc.
733 Third Avenue, New York, NY 10017

© 1982 Ann Bowling and
Ann Cartwright

Typeset by
Scarborough Typesetting Services
and printed in Great Britain at the
University Press, Cambridge

British Library Cataloguing in
Publication Data

Bowling, Ann
    Life after a death.
    1. Bereavement—Psychological aspects
    I. Title   II. Cartwright, Ann
    304.6'4 (expanded)   BF575.G7
    ISBN 0-422-78230-0

Library of Congress Cataloging in
Publication Data

Bowling, Ann.
    Life after a death.
    Bibliography: p.
    Includes indexes.
    1. Widows—England.
    2. Widowers—England.
    3. Aged—England.
    4. Bereavement—Psychological aspects.
    I. Cartwright, Ann.   II. Title.
    HQ1058.5.G7B68   1982   362.8'2
                                            82-8099
    ISBN 0-422-78230-0   AACR2

Contents

home sharers (196) − Future problems (199) − The
feelings of the familiars (200) − The care of the
widowed who were too unfit to take part in our study
(203) − Discussion (211)

10 **What can be done?** 213
The views of the widowed (213) − Some practical
needs (215) − Actions and attitudes of relatives and
friends (220) − The role of the general practitioner
(221) − The role of social and voluntary services (224)
− Summing-up (226)

Appendices

Acknowledgements

A particular debt of gratitude is due to the widows and widowers and their supporters who answered our many questions and recalled many sad and poignant memories to help us. We are grateful to the general practitioners who participated and generously gave us their time.

We would also like to thank the many other people who helped with and contributed to this study:

the interviewers, particularly Pat Amis, Audrey Bassett, Gwen Craddock, Hilary Gellman, Jacquita Glyn, Lesley Hammond, Marjorie Hutchin, Ellen Latham, Nanette Nelson, Gillian Peace, Mollie Richards, Anne Summersby, and Janet York who did most of the interviewing;

the coders, Margaret Hall, Jenny Harding, Alice Hemmings, and Richard Mond;

Alison Britton and Alison Venning who prepared the data for analysis;

Carol Joseph and Danny Kushlick who checked this report;

Michele Becker, Irene Browne, and Christine Fitzgerald who typed the documents and gave administrative support;

Joan Deane, Dorothy Hills, and Lee Drew who punched the cards;

Members of the Institute's Advisory Committee, who supported and advised at various stages: Abe Adelstein, Tony Alment, Val Beral, Vera Carstairs, May Clarke, Geoffrey Hawthorn, Austin

Heady, Margot Jefferys, Joyce Leeson, John McEwan, David
Morrell, Martin Richards, Alwyn Smith, and Michael Wadsworth;

Ivan Hutchinson and Eric Simpson at the Office of Population
Censuses and Surveys, and C. J. Nickless at the Department of
Health and Social Security for their time and resources;

The Department of Health and Social Security who funded the
study and particularly Arthur Forsdick and Marguerite Smith;

The Department of Community Medicine at Manchester University
which gave hospitality.

Among the others who helped in various ways were: Gwen Cartwright, Stephen Hatch, Peter Marris, Colin Murray Parkes, Donald
Patrick, Barry Reedy, Jasper Woodcock, and members of the Institute for Social Studies in Medical Care staff, in particular Robert
Anderson, Madeleine Simms, and Christopher Smith.

1 Introduction

The circumstances in which people are widowed vary from the totally unexpected to the predictable. But once the event has occurred it is clearly labelled so it is a crisis which society can identify. Services and help can be mobilized. This study aims to show the circumstances and ways in which this can most usefully and helpfully be done for elderly widows and widowers. It is the old who are most likely to be widowed and they face this crisis at a time when they may also be adjusting to ill health and increasing infirmity and to retirement with its problems of role identity and adaptation to an increase in leisure and a decrease in wealth. So our survey is about the range of problems which are likely to face the elderly widowed from housing to health, loneliness to lethargy, and penury to the practicalities of day-to-day living.

The difficulties encountered by the elderly widowed will often be similar to those faced by other elderly people: over a third of people aged sixty-five or more are widowed. But around the time of their widowhood they are often confronted by additional problems and decisions. Most will be faced with learning to live alone or uprooting themselves from their home and adjusting to life with relatives. If they choose the latter this will often mean leaving the area where they have been living and their friends and neighbours there. Decisions about which course to adopt may need to be taken in a hurry for financial reasons or because the elderly person needs immediate care and support. Often the elderly person will have been involved in caring for their spouse during his or her terminal illness; this is likely to have been physically and emotionally exhausting but widowhood will mean that they have lost their main occupation and preoccupation. For some, who are themselves disabled, widowhood may mean that they have lost the person who cared for them so that there is an immediate crisis as alternative sources of care need to be found. Others will need to take on the practical and the decision-making tasks previously performed by their spouse. These problems have to be faced in a situation often complicated by the anxiety, loneliness, apathy, and bewilderment of bereavement.

Marris (1974)[1] has described the conflict in adjusting to the death of a close person: the need to adapt to change but also to restore the past.

'Grief . . . is the expression of a profound conflict between contradictory impulses — to consolidate all that is still valuable and important in the past, and to preserve it from loss; and at the same time, to re-establish a meaningful pattern of relationships, in which the loss is accepted. . . . To say that life has lost its meaning is not . . . just a way of expressing apathy. It describes a situation where someone is bereft of purpose and so feels helpless. Familiar habits of thought and behaviour no longer make sense.'

(Marris 1974: 31–3)

In Marris's analysis

'grief is mastered, not by ceasing to care for the dead, but by abstracting what was fundamentally important in the relationship and rehabilitating it. A widow has to give up her husband without giving up all that he meant to her, and this task of extricating the essential meaning of the past and reinterpreting it to fit a very different future, seems to proceed by tentative approximation, momentarily comforting but at first unstable. For a while she may not be able to conceive any meanings in her life except those which are backward-looking and memorial, too tragic to sustain any future. In time, if all goes well, she will begin to formulate a sense of her widowhood, which neither rejects nor mummifies the past, but continues the same fundamental purposes. Until then, she will often be overwhelmed by feelings of disintegration.'

(Marris 1974: 34–5)

This book is concerned with the social setting in which this process takes place and aims to identify some of the factors related to the

[1] References are given in full at the end of the book.

resolution of this conflict. The problems are not only short-term ones. The decisions made in the time immediately after the death will sometimes influence the lives of many people for years ahead. And some decisions are irrevocable. If a home is disbanded and sold it cannot be re-acquired if circumstances prove unsatisfactory.

For the relatives too there will be adjustments and difficult decisions to be made. Faced with competing and conflicting demands — of a widowed parent, a spouse, children, and a job — daughters and sons may be called upon to help and support their widowed parent in his or her decision making while they are also having to resolve their own doubts and difficulties. And the help they give at this stage may be expected to extend indefinitely into the future. So, in addition to identifying the needs of elderly widowed people, describing the ways in which some needs are met and others not, and ascertaining ways in which services could alleviate some of the difficulties, our survey is also concerned with the problems facing the relatives, friends, and neighbours to whom the elderly widowed turn for practical help and emotional support. We look at the perceptions of the people closest to the elderly widowed about the circumstances of the death and the reactions of the widowed to their changed circumstances. This adds another dimension to the picture we have painted since the elderly widowed may sometimes be too apathetic to be aware of some of the things that are happening and too depressed to tell us about the problems they do perceive.

Background to the study

There are a number of social and demographic reasons why elderly widowed people may be given less practical and emotional support from relatives, friends, neighbours, and services now than in the past. First, the proportion living alone has increased: in England and Wales among the widowed or divorced of pensionable age the proportion of men living alone increased from 44% in 1961 to 64% in 1971 and for women from 54% to 69% (Office of Population Censuses and Surveys 1964 and 1975). Secondly increasing mobility (OPCS 1978a) combined with decreasing family size has meant that elderly people not only have fewer children but that their children live further away and ties with neighbours may be less close, partly because they are likely to be shorter. Thirdly increasing employment of women, particularly married women, means that daughters are less available to care for elderly parents when they need help, and neighbours too are likely to have less time and energy to spare. Finally, the increase in the proportion of the population that are elderly together with the emphasis on community rather than institutional care, means that there are increasing demands on already hard-pressed community services.

The problem is probably not that relatives are unwilling to care for elderly people, but that there may not be relatives available to look after them, or sometimes that relatives suffer undue strain in caring for them. This was the conclusion of Isaacs (1971) in a study of the reasons for admission of 280 geriatric patients from their own homes to a geriatric unit in Glasgow. Also, a study of people's lives in the year before they died showed that for widowed, separated, and divorced people the brunt of caring for them was generally borne by relatives, in particular daughters (Cartwright, Hockey, and Anderson 1973).

There have been a number of studies of different parts of the complex and difficult situation faced by widowed people and their supporters. Hinton (1967), Kübler-Ross (1970), Saunders (1966), Wilkes (1965), Glaser and Strauss (1965 and 1968), and others have studied the time before death and the process of dying.

Several authors, including Parkes (1972) and Lindemann (1944) have described distinct phases of bereavement. It typically begins with shock, sometimes accompanied by denial of the death. The next stage identified is a period of intense grief, involving a searching for the lost person, leading to depression and apathy as the loss is accepted. The final stage is one of re-organization and of beginning again. Grief and mourning have been movingly described and studied by Gorer (1965).

Several researchers have looked at mortality following bereavement and found an increase in the year after bereavement: Kraus and Lilienfeld (1959), Young, Benjamin, and Wallis (1963), Rees and Lutkins (1967), and Parkes, Benjamin, and Fitzgerald (1969).

The relatively poor health of widows and their increased use of health services have been described by Maddison and Viola (1968) and Parkes and Brown (1972), while Stein and Susser (1969) showed that the widowed had higher psychiatric hospital admission rates. Macmillan (1963), aware of the increased hospital admission rate among the elderly bereaved, demonstrated that regular calls by a health visitor could achieve a reduction in this rate.

Various factors or circumstances associated with adaptation to bereavement have been identified by Glick, Weiss, and Parkes (1974), Lopata (1973), and Kübler-Ross (1970). Their findings are compared with the results of this study later in the book.

In a number of the studies of the elderly the task of supporting elderly relatives and neighbours has been considered but for most of the studies this has been a relatively peripheral consideration. Those that have looked at this in any depth have shown that relatives take on a major part of the caring for the elderly and infirm and that this can often be a burden and strain physically, emotionally, and socially. Klein, Dean, and Bogdonoff (1967) looking at the impact of illness upon the spouse concluded that the development of illness in the family is attended by role failure which leads to the experience of interpersonal tension and somatic symptoms in both spouses.

None of the studies has looked at the spectrum of problems that confronts both the elderly widowed and their supporters. Marris (1958) looked at the range of problems, social, financial, and emotional faced by young widows but of course the elderly widowed are likely to face additional problems of dependence and ill-health. And those needing extensive support may make heavy demands on their relatives. But, because of the changes mentioned earlier, the elderly widowed are now likely to be rather more dependent on health and social services when they are ill or in need of help. And their most frequent and accessible source of professional help is likely to be their general practitioner (Hunt 1978). So the part played by general practitioners in supporting the elderly widowed is described in some detail in this study and the views of general practitioners on their appropriate role both before and after the death of an elderly married patient are considered.

Methods

The survey was done in eight areas (registration districts or combinations of registration districts) of England, chosen with probability proportional to the number of deaths and taking a random starting point. The way this was done is explained in more detail in Appendix I.

Our aim was to interview the widows of men aged 65 or more and the widowers of women aged 60 or more. The reasons for this are discussed in Appendix II. In each area the Office of Population Censuses and Surveys selected a random sample of 200 deaths that were mostly registered in January 1979.[2] This gave a total sample of 1600 of which just over half were discarded because they were of women under 60 (94 deaths), of men under 65 (256 deaths), or of women aged 60 or more who were not married at the time (513 deaths). The marital status of men who die is not recorded on the non-confidential part of the death certificate, so for male deaths the interviewers' first task was to find out whether or not the men had been married at the time of the death. The sample was found to contain the deaths of 160 married women and 343 married men in the required age groups, a total of 503. This is close to, and certainly well within the range of, the numbers expected from national statistics.

The widows and widowers were visited in their homes from May 1979 onwards. Most of them, 86%, were seen during May, June, or July, that is four to six months after they had been widowed, but some were seen during August, September, and October. The average time was 5.4 months after the death. Fifteen were found to have died since their spouse's death. Of the others 361, 74%, agreed to be interviewed. A further 19, 4%, were too ill or confused to be seen but the person looking after them gave us some limited information about their situation. This is discussed in Chapter 9. Nine, 2%, had moved out of the area or to an address we were unable to trace, but 99, 20%, of the widowed were unwilling to talk to us about their experiences. So the final sample may be biased away from deaths that were particularly upsetting for the widowed. For example one said:

'I'm not ready to discuss anything − it's still too upsetting.'

As data from the death certificates are available for all the deaths in the sample, it is possible to see whether the response varied with the age, sex, and social class of the deceased, or by place, or cause of death, by the person who registered the death, or by area. The only significant difference to emerge was that a higher proportion of widowers than of widows agreed to be interviewed: 83% compared with 70%.[3] Other studies suggest that women find it more difficult than men to adjust to bereavement (see Parkes 1972). So this is a further indication that the failure rate may be high among those most affected.

[2] In one or two areas less than 200 deaths were registered in January, so deaths in the previous month were sampled to make the number up.

[3] Unless otherwise stated attention has not been drawn to differences which might have occurred by chance five or more times in 100.

A third of those who were interviewed cried at some point during the interview and a number indicated that they had found it helpful to talk about their feelings and experiences. One, after a three-and-a-half-hour interview, gave the interviewer a hug and a kiss for having listened to her and commented:

> 'It hasn't really sunk in yet. I think I'm numb. This is the first time I've cried.'

The interviews were generally long ones, partly because we asked a lot of questions but also because interviewers were instructed not to hurry the interview and to let people talk when they wanted to. So half the interviews took between two and three hours, a fifth took less than two hours, and three-tenths three hours or more.[4] Most of the widowed, 78%, were seen on their own.

The doctors

During the course of the interview, the widows and widowers were asked for the name and address of their doctor and 97% (349) gave us this information. Of the twelve who did not, one did not know the doctor's name, one refused, and ten did not complete the interview. All 349 had general practitioners under the NHS, none had a private doctor. A few widows or widowers had the same doctor as others in the sample, so the 349 widowed gave us the names of 295 doctors. All these doctors were traced although five had recently retired and four had moved out of the study area. We also asked the widowed if they were willing for us to ask their doctors about any help and advice the doctor had given to them and for the doctor to give us information about their health and treatment. We explained that we would not tell the doctor anything the widow or widower had said to us. Two hundred and fifty-one of the widowed, 72% of those giving us the name of their doctor, agreed to this and signed a form giving their permission.

We wrote to the 295 general practitioners and sent them a postal questionnaire about their general views and experiences of caring for elderly bereaved people. In addition we sent them 251 questionnaires about individual patients. Eventually 180 (61%) of the general

---

[4] A copy of the questionnaire may be obtained from the Institute for Social Studies in Medical Care, 14 South Hill Park, London, NW3 2SB. There will be a charge for photocopying and postage.

questionnaires were completed and 142 (56%) of the questionnaires about individual patients. This means that we have information from the general practitioner about 39% of the widows and widowers interviewed. These are comparatively low response rates. Can we identify any specific biases?

Data about the date of birth, sex, country of qualification, qualifications, number of partners, type of area, number of patients in the practice, proportion of patients in the practice who were sixty-five and over, and whether or not the doctor was a trainer were available for all the doctors in the sample from the DHSS, and the Royal College of General Practitioners gave us information about their members. This makes it possible to see whether the response rate varied with any of these characteristics. The response rate was relatively high among members of the Royal College of General Practitioners: 76% compared with 58% among non-members to the general questionnaire, and 78% against 52% to the one about individual patients. The only other significant difference to emerge with these basic characteristics was that doctors in practices with an average list size of 3500 or more were less likely to reply to the general questionnaire: 50% compared with 65%.

It is also possible to look at variations in completion rates of doctors with some of the experiences and views of the widowed. General practitioners were more likely to respond if the widow or widower and their spouse went to the same practice, if the widow or widower had consulted their doctor since their spouse died, and if the widow or widower described the care their spouse had received from their general practitioner as 'very good' rather than 'fairly good' or 'not very good'. The figures are in *Table 1*. There was no difference in the completion rate if the spouse died at home or in hospital.

The differences in completion rates among general practitioners could not be explained by variations in the widow's or widower's agreement for the doctors to be approached. Indeed, over one of the characteristics their agreement went in the opposite direction, presumably because of a desire to protect their doctors from further work: the widowed were more likely to agree to us approaching their general practitioner for information about themselves if they regarded their doctor as rather *un*sympathetic — 90% of those widows or widowers agreed, compared with 72% of those who had found him or her very or fairly sympathetic; it was least, 69%, if the widow or widower had not seen their doctor at all since their spouse's death.

Table 1   Some variations in the response of general practitioners with the views and experiences of the widowed

	General practitioner completed general questionnaire	General practitioner completed questionnaire about patient*	Number of widowed (=100%)
Widow or widower and spouse had:			
Same doctor	63%	42%	262
Different doctor in the same partnership	56%	47%	43
Doctor in different practices	48%	24%	46
Widow or widower described general practitioner's care of spouse as:			
Very good	63%	44%	211
Fairly good	54%	33%	79
Not very good	50%	30%	30
Widow or widower described general practitioner as:			
Very sympathetic	69%	48%	148
Fairly sympathetic	55%	38%	47
Rather unsympathetic	33%	24%	21
Widow or widower thought doctor had time to discuss things:			
Yes	64%	47%	265
No	44%	20%	66
Widow or widower consulted own doctor since widowed:			
Five or more times	74%	51%	39
One–four times	61%	43%	192
Not at all	55%	32%	117

* These percentages relate to the proportion of widowed about whom a general practitioner completed a questionnaire (whereas the figures in the text relate to the proportion of dispatched questionnaires that were returned), so part of the 'failure' is due to the widowed not giving their agreement to this part of the study.

In spite of this it seems that doctors who appear understanding and sympathetic to the widowed were more likely to participate in the study.

The familiars

In addition to the general practitioners we asked the widowed to identify the person who knew most about their circumstances at the time of the interview — their 'familiars'.[5] Six per cent did not identify anyone — usually because they did not know anyone closely enough. These widows and widowers were not necessarily those without relatives but those who did not confide in others. One such widow had a daughter whom she saw once a month but said:

> 'No one knows. Well people don't want to know do they? When they ask me at work how I am I always say "I'm alright". I keep cheerful, have a laugh, cover up how I really feel. I'm crying inside really.'

We told the widowed that we would like to get in touch with the person they had mentioned to ask if they would be willing to talk to us. The interviewer explained:

> 'It would not be me so there is absolutely no question of anything you have told me being passed on to him/her. But we would like to explain that we have seen you and that you gave us their name. Of course it would be entirely up to them to say whether they were prepared to help us or not. But we hope that you will be willing to give us their name and address so that we can ask them.'

Four-fifths of them agreed and gave us their full name and address. Those who refused us permission to contact their familiars tended to say that they did not want them bothered. For example:

> 'I don't mind people coming to me but I don't want anyone going to my daughters. I don't want any worries put on them. They have enough worries about me on my own as it is.'

> 'I would rather you didn't trouble her. I wouldn't like her bothered because of me. She's done enough for me already.'

Such comments suggest that some of those who gave more help to the widowed may not have been included in our study.

Eighty-four per cent of the familiars the widowed gave us permission

[5] We did not use this term in the interviews.

to contact were successfully interviewed. This represents two-thirds of those identified by the widowed and means that for 59% of the widows and widowers interviewed we also saw a familiar.

No differences were found between the widowed for whom a familiar was interviewed and those for whom one was not in terms of the widowed person's age, sex, social class, health, or whether they were living alone or with others. The only significant difference was that more of the widowed for whom a familiar was interviewed had children, 89% compared with 75% of the others.

The reasons for interviewing the familiars were two-fold. First, we wanted to find out from their point of view what was involved in being close to an elderly person who had been recently widowed. Secondly we wanted another perspective on the problems facing the elderly widowed. Some people who have experienced a dramatic change in their lives may react by finding subsequent problems overwhelming: set-backs or decisions that they would usually cope with easily may assume Gargantuan proportions or appear insoluble. Others may become numb so that they are almost indifferent to the immediate problems of their day-to-day lives or unaware of the decisions that need to be made. The perspective of another close observer throws some light on the extent and frequency of these different reactions.

The widowed, the general practitioners, and the familiars

So who are the people included in this study? The ages of the widows and widowers are shown in *Table 2*. Widows outnumbered widowers by almost two to one which is to be expected given the basis for our sample. Four widows in our sample were under 55 but none was less than 45. National statistics of the age combinations of married couples at the time that one of them dies (OPCS 1978b) indicate that we would expect 7% of our sample of widows and 4% of our widowers to be under 60. In addition we would expect more of the widowers than of the widows to be 75 or more: 39% compared with 29%. The observed proportions fit in within these expectations.

Two-thirds of the widowed had been married for 40 years or more including a quarter who had had their 50th wedding anniversary and 3% their 60th. Only 7% had been married more than once.

It will sometimes be helpful to make some comparisons of these elderly widows and widowers with people of rather similar ages from the general population. For simplicity they will be compared with

Table 2   Age of the widows and widowers interviewed

	Widows	Widowers	Both sexes
Age group:	%	%	%
Under 55	2	–	1
55–59	6	6	6
60–64	10	11	11
65–69	26	18	23
70–74	28	23	26
75–79	16	23	18
80–84	10	15	12
85–89	1	3	2
90 or more	1	1	1
Number of widowed (= 100%)	226*	124*	350*

* The ages of seven widows and four widowers who did not complete the interview were not obtained. In other tables too small numbers for whom inadequate information was obtained have been excluded.

people aged sixty-five and over in two studies based on samples from the electoral register. The age and sex distribution of the groups that will be compared are shown in *Table 3*. The group of widows and widowers is younger in that it contains 18% who are under 65 but the proportion aged 75 or more is similar in the three groups. There were

Table 3   Age and sex distribution of comparative groups

	The elderly widowed	Cartwright and Anderson (1981)	Dunnell and Cartwright (1972)
Age:	%	%	%
Under 65	18 ⎫ 67	–	–
65–74	49 ⎭	62	69
75 and over	33	38	31
Sex:	%	%	%
Male	35	38	43
Female	65	62	57
Number (= 100%)	361	165	280

* When two or more base numbers are different because of inadequate information the total number has been given.

rather fewer men among the elderly widowed than among those interviewed in the Dunnell and Cartwright study. But the differences are
not large and we have therefore made direct comparisons without
standardization.

The general practitioners

The proportion of single-handed doctors, 20%, was similar to that
among all general practitioners in England, and their age distribution too was roughly comparable. Our sample contained relatively
few female doctors; 9% among those who responded compared with
16% in England generally (DHSS 1980) but this was not because
women were less likely to reply but because comparatively few of the
widowed said they had a woman doctor. In another study (Cartwright
and Anderson 1981) it was also found that women general practitioners had rather younger patients than their male colleagues.
Seventeen per cent of the doctors initially identified were members of
the Royal College of General Practitioners, a similar proportion to
that found by Cartwright and Anderson in 1977 although the College
claims a 25% membership. In both studies College members were
more likely to respond than non-members.

The familiars

Almost half the familiars interviewed, 46%, were daughters, 23%
were sons. Other relatives made up 16%, friends and neighbours
14%. One per cent were professionals. The majority, 69%, were
women.

Summing-up

Starting from a random sample of death certificates of men aged 65
or more and women aged 60 and over in eight randomly selected
areas, 505 widowed people were identified and 361, 74% of them,
were successfully interviewed in their homes, mostly five to six months
after their bereavement. The response rate of 74% is a cause for some
concern. Widows were less likely to agree to be interviewed than
widowers and this adds to the impression that those finding it most
difficult to adjust may have been less willing to be interviewed. The
response rate from the general practitioners of the widowed people

was considerably lower and even more problematic, a number of definite biases being identified. These suggest that the picture portrayed by the general practitioners who did participate may indicate a greater level of involvement and concern with the problems of elderly widowed people than exists among the doctors who did not take part. In addition to the widows and widowers themselves and their general practitioners we also contacted, when the widowed person was willing, the people identified by the widowed as the ones who knew most about their current circumstances.

This three-sided approach enables us to look at the experiences and attitudes of the widowed people themselves, and to consider the implications of the help they got, or sometimes failed to get, from general practitioners and from relatives, friends, and neighbours from the viewpoint of the people involved in giving this support.

2 Caring for the spouse who died

In this chapter we look at the process of becoming widowed. The circumstances leading up to and surrounding the death may determine the extent to which the widow or widower confronts his or her new role in a state of exhaustion, shock, relief, guilt, resignation, indignation, or a combination of these feelings. So we are concerned here with the nature and length of the last illness, the care and support given in the year before death, the widowed person's view of that care, and the impact on his or her life during this time.

The last illness

Widowhood is occasionally a sudden event with no prior warning, but more usually, especially among older people, it is the climax of a period during which life has revolved around caring for a sick spouse. It is the final stage of the role of wife or husband. Indeed for women eventual widowhood can realistically be regarded as a normal part of the process of ageing.

Few, 4%, husbands or wives died suddenly with no previous condition or illness. One was a man of sixty-seven who died suddenly from a heart attack. He had no known previous illness. His widow described what happened:

'We were on the train to Brighton. We got on the train and we had to rush. He put his coat up on the rack and went to pay the fare, he came back and sat bang on the seat. He looked asleep, he gave three quick gasps. The man on the train went to get a doctor. The doctor looked at him and left. I thought "Nobody's doing anything". I tried to undo his tie and rub his chest. They stopped the train at Haywards Heath, they had an awful job to get him out. They got a chair and put him into the ambulance. They gave him oxygen but he was dead. I was in a daze . . . he had just retired twelve weeks before and we were going to spend our time at the caravan. We had just bought a caravan at Peacehaven.'

Two-fifths of the widowed said the death was expected as far as they were concerned.[1] An illustration of such a death is:

'He was treated for two years with gastro-enteritis and pains in his back. He had primary cancer in his stomach and spleen − he had them removed but it had gone too far. The doctors gave him two months but I kept him alive by nursing him for eighteen months, and they sent me no nursing help at all.'

Coping with illness over a long period may make the surviving spouse tired and, if they do not get adequate support, resentful. But it can give them an opportunity to prepare for the changes ahead. One widower commented that he had few problems now as he had had time to prepare himself for the death and adjust to new roles:

'No problems really. If she'd gone suddenly it would have been much more of a blow.'

Just over half, 56%, of the deaths were neither completely instantaneous nor expected from the point of view of the spouse who survived. The person had been ill but was not expected to die or to die then. A widow whose husband had had back trouble for nine years and died of a heart attack describes one such death:

'About twelve months before his death he had a pain in his leg. The GP said it was hardening of the arteries. He got no better so had a letter to go into hospital. When he got there he had a complete examination − X-rays, the lot. The hospital found a spot on his lung and he was admitted for nine days for further tests. He felt

---

[1] A series of questions were asked about this: 'What did he/she die of?'; 'Did he/she have any other illness or condition?'; 'Could you say how long —— was ill before he/she died?'. IF NOT AT ALL: (a) 'So did he/she die instantaneously?'; (b) 'And was he/she completely fit before he/she died?'; 'So would you say ——'s death was expected or not as far as you were concerned?'.

perfectly allright all the time except for his leg. The specialist didn't tell either of us what was the matter but said he must have an operation on his lung. We thought it was just for the spot. He wouldn't have it done before Christmas — didn't really want it anyway but the specialist said if you don't have it done you may only live another six months. If you do have it you could live another ten to fifteen years. That decided him. He said he wanted all those extra years with me. Nobody mentioned cancer to either of us. I can't forgive them not telling me. I learnt it right at the end from the GP — just before the op. She thought I knew — said the specialist should have been the one to tell me.'

Expected deaths were, not surprisingly, rather more common among older people aged 85 or more: the proportion was 65% for them compared with 39% of deaths of younger people; a finding supported by Cartwright, Hockey, and Anderson (1973). There was no trend with age among those under 85. Expected deaths were also more common if the cause was cancer,[2] 56%, or bronchitis, or other respiratory diseases, 53%; whereas it was 34% for deaths from other causes. And, as might be predicted, the death was more often expected if the person had been ill for a long time: it was expected for 49% of those who had been ill for two years or more in comparison with 31% of those who had been ill for a shorter period.[3] The length of time the person was said to have been ill is shown in *Table 4*.[4] There was no significant variation with the sex of the deceased and little variation, among this group of older people, with age. Roughly a third were ill for less than a year, a third for between one and five years, and a third for longer.

It was not only the length but also the nature of the illness which contributed to the distress of both the person who died and the surviving spouse. A symptom which gave rise to much concern and anguish for their relatives was confusion. Just under a third, 30%, of the deceased were said by the widowed to have been mentally confused before they died. The length of time they had been confused and the variation in this with the sex of the deceased is shown in *Table 5*. Although women were not significantly more likely than men to have

[2] For a classification of cause of death see Appendix V.
[3] When the deceased had been acutely ill for a short period but chronically ill for longer, we took the longer period.
[4] 'Could you say how long —— was ill before he/she died?'

Table 4   Length of illness

	All deaths
	%
Not ill at all	5
Less than a month	9
1 month but less than 6 months	12
6 months but less than 1 year	5
1 year but less than 2 years	8
2 years but less than 5 years	24
5 years but less than 10 years	14
10 years or more	23
Number of deaths (= 100%)	358

Table 5   Variation in confusion with sex

	Sex of deceased		Both sexes
	Male	Female	
Length of time *confused before death:*	%	%	%
Not at all	73	66	70
Less than a week	6	5	5
1 week but less than 1 month	7	6	7
1 month but less than 3 months	4	3	4
3 months but less than 6 months	2	5	3
6 months but less than 1 year	4	5	5
A year or more	4	10	6
Number of deaths (= 100%)	232	126	358

been described as confused, more of the women had been confused
for six months or more.

Almost two-thirds, 63%, of the widowed whose spouses were
mentally confused found this 'very distressing', and 12% found it
'fairly distressing'. Three descriptions were:

'He used to have brain storms, at least that's what I'd call them
because he tried to strangle me a couple of times and he said he was
going to poison me; he knew how to do it.'

'He used to lose his way home, and one day he moved all the dandelions from the side alley and planted them in the front garden. He didn't know. I had bad nerves and I used to lean on him, but when he became so ill I had to be the one to do everything. I used to send him to the shop with a piece of paper but people said I shouldn't send him any more – he used to forget where the shop was. In the end I wouldn't let him go.'

'She wouldn't know me or her sister at times and she'd order me out of the house. She used to walk about with £15 in her shoes and she'd wander round and people would ring me up and tell me. She'd excrete in the bath and sometimes it would be on her hands. I had to see she'd washed her hands properly. Then she'd lose money and rings and say I'd pinched them. Sometimes she'd put her knickers on her head and she'd get all her dresses out of the wardrobe at night.'

As expected, confusion was relatively often reported for those dying of cerebrovascular accidents, two-fifths. More surprisingly, it was more common for people dying in their seventies, 35%, than for those in their sixties, 23%, or eighties, 22%.

Two-fifths of the widowed said the deceased had other symptoms or problems which they themselves had found distressing. These included pain, depression, sleeplessness, incontinence, inability to move, vomiting, loss of appetite, difficulty breathing or talking, and difficulty eating or feeding.

'He couldn't hold his knife to eat. Things kept shooting off his plate.'

'Vomiting all the time. He was all dirty and my daughters used to clean him up, all sick and blood.'

So widowhood for most, three-quarters, was preceded for a period of six months or more when their spouse was ill, and this was often accompanied by distressing symptoms. What help did they get during that time? The extent of hospital care is considered first.

Care in the last year

Married people are less likely than single or widowed people to die in hospital (see Cartwright, Hockey, and Anderson 1973); but the proportion of all deaths occurring in hospital is gradually increasing: in 1966 54% were in hospitals or 'other institutions for the care of the sick' (General Register Office 1967), by 1977 this proportion had risen to 60% (OPCS 1979). Just over half, 53%, of the deaths in our sample

Table 6   Length of time in hospital or other institution during the last year of life

| | Those dying: | | All sample |
	In hospital or institution	At home or elsewhere	
	%	%	%
Not at all	–	57	26
Less than a week	32	7	20
1 week but less than 1 month	31	15	24
1 month but less than 3 months	24	19	22
3 months but less than 6 months	6	2	4
6 months but less than 1 year	4	–	2
All year	3	–	2
Number of deaths (= 100%)	190	162	352

took place in hospital. In addition, 44% of those dying at home were admitted to hospital at some time during the last year of their lives, so altogether three-quarters, 74%, of these married people spent some part of their last year in hospital. But few were there for long. Only a small minority, 8%, had spent three months or longer in hospital. The figures are in *Table 6*.

Those who had been ill for between three months and two years were *more* likely to have been in hospital than those who had been ill for two years or more. This is shown in *Table 7*. Presumably people are more likely to be admitted in the early stages of an illness; then, after investigations, they are discharged home. Clearly most caring takes place at home. Further evidence to support this comes from an analysis by age. Those aged eighty or more at the time of their death were the ones *least* likely to have been in a hospital or institution in the year before they died: 55% compared with 77% of younger people.

The wives were more likely than the husbands to have died in a hospital or institution − 61% in comparison with 49%; in addition more of the wives had spent a month or more of the last year of their lives in a hospital or institution − 40% against 24% of the husbands. It might be thought that these differences arose because women were more willing to care for their spouses at home but we could not find any clear evidence that this was so.

Table 7 Length of time in hospital or other institution in the year before death by length of illness

	Length of illness					
	Less than a week	1 week < 3 months	3 months < 1 year	1 < 2 years	2< 5 years	5 years or more
Length of time in hospital or institution	%	%	%	%	%	%
Not at all	65	28	6	14	25	26
Less than a week	35	23	14	17	25	15
1 week but less than 1 month	–	34	33	35	20	23
1 month but less than 3 months	–	15	28	28	23	26
3 months but less than 1 year	–	–	19	3	6	7
A year or more	–	–	–	3	1	3
Number of deaths (=100%)	31	39	36	29	84	130

Those who were mentally confused were more likely to have spent some time in a hospital or another institution in the last year of their lives; 90% against 67% of those who were not described as confused. The proportion who were confused increased from 12% of those who had not been in hospital at all to 29% of those who had spent less than a week there, 35% of those who had spent between a week and three months of the last year of their lives in hospital, and 61% of those in for three months or longer. It is obviously impossible to disentangle cause and effect in this relationship.

Those who died of cancer or whose death was attributed to pneumonia or influenza were more likely to have spent some time in hospital than those dying of other causes. (This is shown in *Table 8*.) A comparatively high proportion of the cancer deaths occurred among people under 70, 49% compared with 29% of deaths from other causes, whereas among the deaths ascribed to pneumonia or influenza there was a high proportion of people aged 80 or over, 31% against 13% for other causes. *Table 8* also shows the relationship of the recorded cause of death to the length of time the person had been ill. Half of those who died of bronchitis were said by their surviving husband or wife to have been ill for at least ten years, but none had spent as much as half their last year in hospital. Deaths from

Table 8 Cause of death by length of time in hospital or institution in the year before death and by length of illness

	Cause of death						
	Malignant neoplasm	*Ischaemic heart disease*	*Cerebrovascular accident*	*Other circulatory disease*	*Pneumonia or influenza*	*Bronchitis*	*Other*
Length of time in hospital or institution:	%	%	%	%	%	%	%
Not at all	10	42	28	34	6	29	19
Less than a week	16	20	23	16	21	32	23
1 week but less than 1 month	38	19	20	19	18	21	23
1 week but less than 3 months	28	13	23	28	31	14	23
3 months but less than 6 months	4	2	3	3	9	4	9
6 months but less than 1 year	3	2	3	–	9	–	–
A year or more	1	2	–	–	6	–	3
Length of illness:	%	%	%	%	%	%	%
Not at all	–	11	8	3	3	–	–
Less than a week	–	4	8	9	3	4	8
1 week but less than 1 month	4	4	5	9	9	4	4
1 month but less than 3 months	10	6	3	6	–	7	4
3 months but less than 6 months	11	2	8	6	6	–	8
6 months but less than 1 year	12	4	7	3	–	–	4
1 year but less than 2 years	11	9	8	6	11	–	4
2 years but less than 5 years	23	23	25	21	23	19	34
5 years but less than 10 years	15	15	13	12	20	15	11
10 years or longer	14	22	15	25	25	51	23
Number of deaths (= 100%)	81	114	39	33	35	28	31

bronchitis and from ischaemic heart disease were the ones most likely to occur at home (64% and 50% respectively) while deaths ascribed to pneumonia and influenza were least likely to do so (17%). Many of those in this last category will have been ill with other conditions before developing pneumonia or influenza. The proportion who had been ill for five years or more was lowest for people dying from malignant neoplasms or cerebrovascular accidents and it was ischaemic heart disease and cerebrovascular accidents which had the highest proportion of quick deaths.

The extent to which general practitioners were involved in the care of these married people in the year before they died is shown in *Table 9.* Just over two-fifths, 42% had ten or more consultations with a general practitioner in the year before they died, and almost three out of ten, 29%, had ten or more home visits. In terms of numbers of

Table 9 General practitioner consultations and home visits before death

	General practitioner consultations			General practitioner home visits		
	Place of death			Place of death		
	Hospital or institution	Own home	All deaths*	Hospital or institution	Own home	All deaths*
Number in twelve months before death:	%	%	%	%	%	%
None**	10	4	8	20	15	18
One	8	7	7	14	9	13
Two–four	22	20	21	25	25	24
Five–nine	21	24	22	16	15	16
Ten or more	39	45	42	25	36	29
Number of deaths (=100%)	192	149	359	193	145	356

  * Includes 18 people dying in other places.
 ** Includes 6 people (i.e. 3% of hospital deaths and 2% of all deaths) who were in a hospital or institution for twelve months before they died.

consultations those dying at home appeared to receive only marginally more care from their general practitioners in the last year than those who died in hospital. And those who had spent some time of the last year of their lives in hospital had if anything rather more contact with their general practitioners. The estimated average number of general practitioner consultations rose from 6.6 for those who had not been in hospital at all to 8.7 for those in hospital for more than a month.

Those dying from cancer and from bronchitis were the ones who had most contact with their general practitioners both in terms of total consultations and home visits. (The figures for the proportion with ten or more consultations were: 56% of those dying of cancer, 54% of deaths ascribed to bronchitis, 36% for other causes of death; then the proportion with ten or more home visits: 41% for cancer deaths, 44% deaths for bronchitis, 23% other causes.) Those who had been confused had no more nor less contact with their general practitioners than those who had not. So it would seem that those dying from cancer got relatively more care from both hospitals and general practitioners, while those dying from bronchitis got more care from the general practitioner and relatively little care from hospitals, and the confused were more likely to be looked after in hospital.

Turning to the help they needed while at home it can be seen from *Table 10* that nearly half of all those who died had needed help while at home with dressing or undressing and a similar proportion with bathing, while two-fifths had needed some help at night. A relatively high proportion of those dying from cancer, 80%, and those whose deaths were ascribed to pneumonia or influenza, 79%, had needed some sort of help while at home. And *Table 10* also shows the heavy demands of those who had been confused.

Table 10 Care at home by whether or not the person had been mentally confused at all before death

	Mentally confused before death		All deaths
	Yes	No	
Type of care given:	%	%	%
Dressing and undressing	65	38	46
Getting in or out of bath	64	39	47
Washing or shaving	53	35	41
Being lifted	65	34	43
Getting to lavatory	60	32	41
Help or care at night	61	33	42
Other care of this sort	28	15	19
None	18	42	35
Number of deaths (= 100%)	106	252	359

In over a third of instances where any help was given, 38%, the widowed person had done everything, and in a further third, 39%, they had helped mainly. For 17% the care was equally shared between the widowed and others, and for 6% the care was given mainly or entirely by people other than the widowed. There was no difference between the widows and the widowers who said this care had fallen mainly or entirely on them. Apart from the spouse the main person who gave help when it was needed was a relative, 31%, a professional person, 25%, and a friend or neighbour, 6%. A fifth of the widowed felt that their spouse or they themselves could have done with more help; help with lifting being the most frequent need, by one in eight.

The burden on those widowed who had cared mainly or entirely for their spouses often seemed considerable:

'I had yards of washing as I made pads — he didn't like water-proofs. The nurse said it was my own fault as he wouldn't use a bottle but was happier with the towels.'

'He had a stroke three years ago. It left him paralysed and he never spoke afterwards. He was like a baby. I managed to look after him all the time. He was able to use the one leg if I helped him to. He got gradually worse. Finally, he went into hospital on Friday and died on the Tuesday. . . . I would get him out into the sun sometimes. It was a struggle but I did it. In fact I dropped him several times when I had to lift him, he was ten stone!'

What did the widowed feel about the way their spouses had been looked after during this time?

Attitudes to care

The widowed were asked what they felt about the care and treatment their spouse had from their general practitioner before their death and then to sum up whether this care was 'very good', 'fairly good', or 'not very good'. We have already noted that 8% had no contact with a general practitioner in the year before their death. For the others, in two-thirds the care was felt to be 'very good', a quarter of the widowed described it as 'fairly good', and a tenth as 'not very good'. Comments illustrate the things they appreciated or felt critical about. First in relation to visiting:

'I was highly satisfied with our doctor − he never refused to turn out once, and they've come at all times − during the night and everything.'   (Very good)

'He could have come more often. I was coping allright so they didn't come. It was 24-hour constant attendance for me.'

(Not very good)

'Bar the last week it was very good. I still don't understand why they didn't come then − perhaps because he was going into a coma. Doctors don't seem to give the care they used to. They only seem to care for the crease in their pants and how they dress.'   (Very good)

'I think he could have done better. He grumbled at me for calling the emergency doctor out and said it would cost him £6. I said I would pay for it.'   (Not very good)

Then about the information they were given:

'He got marvellous treatment. They were very, very kind. They didn't tell any lies. They didn't cover anything up. I wanted to be told the truth.'

'They couldn't have been kinder. I think they knew but they wouldn't tell me.'

'Nobody told me about the allowance you can get [the attendance allowance] no-one talked to me or anything. He had to have a special diet of fish and Complan because of his stomach. It cost me a lot of money, but no-one helped.'   (Not very good)

And about the diagnosis or treatment:

'I think her own doctor could have given her more attention and I told him so. If he had taken more time to examine her two years earlier, when she first complained, they might have found the cancer and been able to do something about it.'   (Fairly good)

Other praise and criticism was more general:

'They couldn't have been better if they'd been the King's doctors. They didn't run in and out — they stayed while he wanted them.'
(Very good)

'I expect it was OK. That doesn't mean I agree with what doctors do these days. I used to think they were dedicated people but I don't think that now. In fact I feel quite angry about doctors in general but not particularly in relation to my husband's death.'
(Fairly good)

'I have no confidence in him. He's allright with young ones, he has no time for old ones, he can't be bothered with us.'
(Not very good)

The widows' and widowers' views of the way general practitioners looked after their husband or wife did not differ significantly with the place or cause of death, nor with age or sex of the person who died. But those whose spouse had been seen ten or more times by a general practitioner were more likely to describe the care as very good, 74% of them did so compared with 57% of those whose husband or wife was seen less often. The picture in relation to visits is similar; here the relatively satisfied were those whose spouse had had five or more visits: 77% of them described the care as 'very good' compared with 52% of the others.

Assessments of care were also clearly related to social class.[5] Those in Social Classes I and II were most likely to describe the care as

[5] For the classification of social class see Appendix IV.

'very good' and those in Classes IV and V were least likely to feel this. The figures are in *Table 11*. Is this because those in Social Classes I and II received better attention from their doctors? There was no evidence from this study that they had more consultations or more home visits. But other studies (Buchan and Richardson 1973; Cartwright and O'Brien 1976) have found that general practitioners spend rather longer talking to their middle-class than to their working-class patients.

Table 11   Social class and views of the widowed on the way the general practitioner looked after their husband or wife

	Social class of husband's occupation					All classes**
	I and II Professional & Intermediate	III (N) Skilled Non-manual	III (M) Skilled manual	IV Semi-skilled	V Unskilled	
Assessment of general practitioner care:	%	%	%	%	%	%
Very good	82	64	64	56	55	65
Fairly good	12	22	23	33	33	24
Not very good	6	8	9	11	12	9
Other comment	–	6	4	–	–	2
Number of widowed (=100%)*	49	36	142	64	33	327

* Those who had not seen their general practitioner in the year before they died have been excluded.
** Includes three who could not be classified by social class.

On balance the widowed were slightly less critical of the care their spouses had received from the hospital than from their general practitioners. Nearly three-quarters of those whose spouse had been in hospital felt their care and treatment there had been 'very good'. Those who assessed the care their spouse had had from a general practitioner as 'very good' were more likely to regard their hospital care also as 'very good' than those who were at all critical of the general practitioner care. This can be seen from *Table 12*.

One reason for the association might be people's different expectations and standards. Another one could be that some people regard the organization of a referral to good hospital care as part of their general practitioner's job. If the general practitioner sent their husband or wife to a hospital which did not look after them well, then this might be counted against the general practitioner. Obviously not

Table 12 Relationship between widows' and widowers' assessments of general practitioner and hospital care of spouse

	Assessment of general practitioner care:			All those receiving hospital care
	Very good	Fairly good	Not very good	
Assessment of hospital care:	%	%	%	%
Very good	82	64	57	73
Fairly good	10	27	35	18
Not very good	5	6	8	6
Other comment	3	3	–	3
Number of widowed (=100%)	170	63	26	286

all the widowed felt that way since over half those who rated their spouse's hospital care as 'not very good' described the care they had from the general practitioner as 'very good'. A third possibility is that people who are skilled at obtaining good care from one source are likely to be better at getting it from another source too. But in relation to social class, assessments by the widowed of their spouse's care in hospital went, if anything, in the opposite direction from their assessment of general practitioner care. Fewer of the middle-class widowed described it as very good (62% compared with 76% of the working-class widowed) – but there was no clear trend, nor was there any social class difference in the proportion opting for 'not very good'. The higher expectations of the middle-class may not be met by a correspondingly better service in hospital.

The level of distress experienced by the few who had poor, or no, care from both general practitioner and hospital is illustrated by one widow who had nursed her husband (who died of lung cancer) for over four years. She had given up her work, visiting friends, or going out for any social activities. She had not had a holiday and she had stopped entertaining people at home:

'I'd rush out to do the shopping and back home again.'

Her husband had not seen a general practitioner at all in the year before he died although he'd been at home for more than half that time. She said the doctor would not come when she telephoned, he always sent for an ambulance. Her husband had four spells in hospital during the last year of his life and eventually died there. Describing his care in hospital she said:

'They would not allow us to visit him − only visiting hours − although they knew he was dying. He was screaming with pain and they couldn't help him. He was a clean man, yet he was always covered in sick and blood when we called. It was awful when he screamed.'

She had not been told he had cancer:

'I had asked the doctors. They wouldn't tell me anything. I could see it must be more than just heart − but they wouldn't say.'

We asked the widowed whose spouses died at home whether they would rather the person had been in hospital or whether they were glad he or she had died at home. The majority, 91%, said they were glad their spouse had been at home when he or she died:

'I'm glad he was in his own home and I was there.'

Among the five who said outright that it would have been better if the person had been in hospital were two who were somewhat critical of their general practitioners:

'They didn't bother with him. I don't suppose they could do much for him. They were very nice, but they're busy aren't they? I didn't dare send for him. He came once and said "There's nothing I can do for him". We couldn't lift him. He was a dead weight − even the nurse said it was too much. It used to be terrible. She said he ought to be in hospital in a special bed. He had terrible back sores. They did their best to get him into hospital.'

'They should have sent him to hospital in my opinion. He [general practitioner] only gave him tablets. I should have pushed the doctor more to send him to hospital. They should have put him on a heart machine. I've been twice on a heart machine for check-up.' (Husband died of heart attack. Had had angina for two or three months.)

Another widow thought the hospital had sent her husband home too soon, while another just thought her husband would have been looked after better in hospital.

We also asked the widowed whose spouses died in hospital whether, if adequate nursing and other help had been available, it would have been possible for the deceased to have been looked after at home. The majority, 82%, said 'no'. The main reason given by four-fifths of these, was that hospital facilities were needed. Of the 18% who said it would have been possible for the deceased to have been looked after at home, almost half still said it was better that the deceased was in hospital, but 9% would have preferred to have had them at home. A third of these were critical of the way their spouses had been looked after in hospital.

One widower, when asked what his wife died of said:

'A broken heart I think, but at the hospital they told me she had a shrunken bladder. They should never have taken her away. I should never have let them persuade me.'

When his wife went blind two years before her death, she had gone into a geriatric hospital.

'When they get you into hospital they make you sit in a chair for hours, then you progress to a wheel chair and from there to an infection and that's it. Old people should never be allowed to die like that. They should be kept with the family unit.' (On the death certificate the cause of death was given as bronchopneumonia and cerebral arteriosclerosis.)

Another woman had been in a general hospital for three months and then a geriatric one for four months before she died. Her widower said:

'I felt she could have had better nursing. They could have been a little kinder I felt. She didn't seem to be happy. They didn't speak to her right.'

A man who had also been in a geriatric hospital but for just a month was described by his widow as not being happy there.

'He wasn't happy there and didn't like their attitude. He could have been mentally ill I suppose but he felt they didn't want to be bothered with him. I would have preferred to nurse him. I've nursed a number of people until they died but my husband was a dead weight and I couldn't lift him. If I'd had help with the lifting I could have had him home. I asked at the Civic Centre if there was lifting apparatus available but they said only for long-term cases.'

Kalish and Reynolds (1976) found that most people prefer to die at home and that their relatives are also glad when deaths occur at home rather than in hospital. But in our study, for both home and hospital deaths, the great majority of the widowed, nine-tenths, felt they had happened in the most appropriate place. Rather similar findings in relation to place of birth came from another study (Cartwright 1979). In general people seem reluctant to express a wish that circumstances had been different. When we asked the widowed whether there was anything they wished could have been done differently before their spouse died[6] the majority, three-quarters, said 'no', but a significant minority, almost a quarter, said there was something. This proportion was similar for home and hospital deaths.

When asked what they would have liked done differently most of their replies related to the care given to the deceased − 44% of the answers were concerned with this and most were complaints about the medical or nursing care:

'[I wish] they'd sent him to hospital sooner. Mind you, things were in a bad way − strikes and that. I suppose they didn't want to admit people if they could help it. When I told the doctor I couldn't manage him any longer because of his dead weight, he said if I sent him to hospital "it would be geriatric and you wouldn't like that". I could have done with help from the district nurses too. In the end the doctor did arrange for them to call. His receptionist made the call too late for them to come that day though. I got stuck with my husband half in and half out of bed, so I rang them up and they said they couldn't manage to come that day. When they did arrive, he was in hospital.'

'Better if he'd [doctor] made the right diagnosis. He said it was a virus. . . . She screamed about the pain in her head. Her face was on fire. The doctor said she's picked up a bug and not to give her anything to eat.' (Cause of death: coronary artery occlusion.)

'I would have liked to know whether they could have eased his pain for him. His mouth was like a flame of fire. A bit more treatment.'

'The doctor coming quicker. They should have been able to tell she was serious enough to die.'

'I feel if he'd gone to [a different] hospital he'd still be here.'

[6] 'Taken all together, how do you feel about the way things went before —— died − is there anything you wish could have been done differently?'

These complaints may have reflected genuine dissatisfactions but some may have arisen from the anger, a recognized stage of bereavement, in which perceptions are distorted in the need to blame someone for the death. Parkes (1970) found such anger, often involving a feeling of guilt, to be typical in the early stages of grief. In particular, anger about delay or failure in diagnosis was common. Parkes also reported that seeking for someone to blame, usually the doctor, the hospital, or themselves for the death, was characteristic of this period. Doctors are an obvious target for these feelings – they have failed to prevent the death so it may be felt that they have 'allowed' it to take place.

Marris (1974) argues that widowhood is a time when relationships are anxiously re-examined in an attempt to seek reassurance that everything was done that could have been done to make the dying person happy. Reassurance from doctors or nurses about this seemed to play an important part in preventing or reducing feelings of guilt or anger. People who said that there was nothing that they wish could have been done differently often commented that the medical and nursing staff had done all they could:

'They couldn't have done anything different.'

'I understand that everything was done that could be done for her.'

Parkes (1972) reported that 13 of the 22 London widows in his sample expressed ideas of self-reproach. He argued:

'A major bereavement shakes confidence in (our) sense of security. The tendency to go over events leading up to the loss and to find someone to blame even if it means accepting blame oneself is a less disturbing alternative than accepting that life is uncertain. If we can find someone to blame or some explanation that will enable death to be evaded, then we have a chance of controlling things.'
(Parkes 1972:107)

And we found that 8% of the widowed people answering our question about things they wished had been done differently described regrets about their relationship with the deceased, often expressing self-reproach:

'I've often wondered if I'd done enough.'

'I wish I had retired when he packed up work and spent more time with him.'

A further 4% said they wished the deceased had sought medical care earlier and these often said they wished they had made the deceased seek help:

'If she'd gone earlier to the doctor. I feel sorry that I didn't make her go.'

'I wish I had made him go to the doctor sooner. He didn't want to go although I could see he wasn't looking too well.'

Four per cent said they wished they had spoken more about the death:

'To say "Goodbye". To say something.'

Five per cent wished they had stayed with the deceased longer, or been there at the death:

'My one wish, the only wish, that I could have been there when he died.'

'That I'd stayed with him at the last. But I didn't want to be a nuisance to my neighbours and they were waiting for me. Mrs —— said "let's have a cup of tea and come back" but I said "no". I couldn't expect them to wait for me. I hardly knew them.'

Ten per cent wanted more information about the illness or death or wished they had known about the impending death:

'I just wish we had known about the ulcer – he could have had an operation then.'

'I only wish they'd told me [she had cancer]. If I'd known we would have spoken ordinary, and I would have liked to have talked to her about it. But I didn't know.'

'I wish they would have explained it to me more fully at the hospital. They didn't really help me at all there. They could have explained more what the trouble was and what really happened.'

Finally, 4% said they wished their domestic arrangements had been different (for example, better heating) and 4% said they wished the death had taken place at home. Eleven per cent gave various other replies, for example about the circumstances of the death, the cold weather at the time and about their own health.[7]

The proportion who would have liked something done differently

---

[7] Figures do not add up to 100% as four people gave more than one type of response.

was higher, 39%, if the general practitioner had never visited their spouse at home in the last year, compared with 21% when he or she had done so. And their reactions over this were clearly related to their assessment of the care received: the proportion who wished something could have been done differently rose from 14% of those who described the general practitioner's care of their spouse as 'very good' to 53% of those who felt it was 'not very good'.

However, some of the widowed expressed criticisms with the care given, despite favourable general evaluations. For example, one widow who said the care and treatment the general practitioner had given the deceased was 'very good' also said:

> 'This doctor is very abrupt, he used to upset us and he used to shout at him. He'd ask him something and he didn't give him time to answer. He told my brother "I think he's putting it on". I'll say he's a good doctor but he upsets his patients.'

Another widower who said the hospital care his wife had received was 'very good' had said:

> 'When I saw the condition she came home in I was surprised. She went away all right and came home with bed sores.'

A tendency to express general satisfaction with health services has been found in many other studies. Elderly people in particular seem reluctant to express dissatisfaction. Possibly this is because they remember what it was like before there was a National Health Service, or perhaps they are hesitant about criticizing because they feel more dependent on services.

Feeling that they were left to look after their dying spouse on their own without adequate support clearly contributed to a wish that things had been done differently. Just over a third, 35%, of those whose personal care of the deceased had been left entirely to them would have liked something to have been done differently, compared with a fifth of those who had at least some help with this, and a similar proportion, a fifth, of those whose spouse had not needed such care. How did looking after their husband or wife affect their lives?

Restrictions on the surviving spouse

Some of the widowed had been under a great deal of strain in caring for their ill spouse. The following examples are of widows who cared for their husbands entirely on their own. They both said they could have done with help:

> 'He wasn't able to get into a bath. I used to have to wash him all down. He couldn't even stand in the shower for that length of time. I had to lift him up the bed. He used to pull the door and hang onto the door-handle and I'd help him up.'

> 'I was exhausted when he passed away after looking after him. The nurse promised to bring me a stool so I could put it on the bath. She kept promising but they never came. They sent a night commode but that was only suitable for a lady. My husband was fifteen stone, he couldn't sit on it.'

Also, many of those who said no help, or no more help, was needed with caring for their husband or wife went on to say that this was because they would not have accepted help from anyone other than the widow or widower.

> 'He didn't want to be exposed to the nurses, he was a modest sort of man.'

> 'He didn't want anyone else to do things for him – it's private and personal. I used to rush my shopping so I could get back to him. I had not had a full night's sleep for eighteen months.'

> 'I don't believe he wanted anybody to do anything for him except me. I was getting worse in myself. I couldn't cope. I hadn't been outside the door for two months.'

> 'Well it didn't do me any good. I was worried to death. I had no social life at all and I had no holiday. He was a very shy person and I used to do the things for him because he didn't want anyone else.'

Similarly, one of the familiars commented that the deceased had preferred his spouse to help with nursing care as he found personal help from others embarrassing:

> 'He would get embarrassed, with me being his daughter, and wouldn't let me help except at the very end. The night he died he let me clean him. He said "Fancy you having to do this". Ten minutes later it was the end.'

Even when professional nursing care was given the widowed sometimes commented that it was inadequate because it was hurried or infrequent. In one case the nurse came just fortnightly to bath the deceased, and in another the nurses visited but asked relatives to help as they had such little time:

> 'We had a very hard time. My daughter and I had to help him with everything at the end − eating and everything. My daughter helped so much with him − she washed him, cleaned him. The nurses came every day but they were often in a rush so they often used to ask my daughter to take over. She would do anything.'

We asked the widowed if they had given up or done less of anything during the time of the deceased's illness. Thirty-six per cent had not, more, 53%, had given up something, and 11% had done less of something. The activities they cut down on were: visiting friends or relatives for 45% of all the widowed; going out to other social activities, 46%; going on holiday, 41%; entertaining people at home, 31%; going to work, 12%. Restrictions on other activities were mentioned by 10%.

A quarter, 26%, said their activities were 'severely restricted', and a fifth, 19%, said they were 'fairly restricted'. Another fifth, 21%, said they were 'a little restricted' and for a third, 34%, there was no restriction on activities at all. Many of those who said their activities were not, or only a little, restricted, said this was because they had no outside activities to be disrupted. For example:

> 'Social wise we never went out anyway, so that didn't matter.'

The strain imposed by caring for the dying spouse was greater when the surviving husband or wife was not robust. The proportion who said their activities had been severely restricted increased from 21% of those who rated their own health as excellent or good, to 31% of those who rated it as fair, and 44% of those who regarded it as poor. It was not that those in poor health were more likely to have given up visiting relatives or friends, or entertaining people at home, but that they apparently became too exhausted to do even ordinary activities. One widow said:

> 'I was an ill person over eighty with a heart complaint and yet they sent a dying man home to me with no help at all. I had a bed downstairs for him but he was always messing it. He had no control over his legs. When he fell I had a twelve stone man to lift − and I've got a heart condition! I was so tired my ankles were enormous at night. I had to sleep in the chair in the end as I was too tired to go up and down stairs.'

Restrictions on the activities of the spouse were rather greater for cancer deaths than for others. Thirty-six per cent of the widowed whose spouse had died of cancer said their activities had been severely restricted compared with 23% of other deaths. At the same time the longer the illness the more likely it was to restrict the spouse's activities: 53% of those whose spouse was ill for less than six months had been restricted in some way, compared with 65% when the illness lasted between six months and two years, and 76% for longer illnesses.

The more restricted their lives had been the more likely the widowed were to wish something could have been done differently. The proportion wishing this rose from 18% of those who were not restricted to 33% of the severely restricted.

Those whose spouses died in hospital were somewhat less likely to have given up or done less of something, 62%, than those whose spouses died at home, 74%:

'I couldn't go far. I couldn't go anywhere — just down the road, shopping. I couldn't leave him for any length of time. It made me confused and ill at times — looking after him for so long. For the past few months I had to carry him to the bathroom.'

'I didn't go out — it caused my blood pressure. I used to like a drink at the pub but I couldn't leave her, or ask anyone to stop in whilst I went for a drink. You can't do that can you?'

In addition to restrictions on physical activities, the widowed often mentioned the mental strain they suffered in the period before the death:

'It was nerve-racking   living with the knowledge that he could die any day. When he was choking I was on my own and there was no-one to help me — I never saw a nurse. I had to be awake at night because of the choking. I wasn't give any advice as to what to do for him.' (Died from cancer of the stomach.)

'You think "what's going to happen to him?". You're tensed up all the time.'

Widows and widowers of spouses described as mentally confused before the death were more likely to say their activities had been 'severely restricted' at that time, 39% compared with 20% of the widowed whose spouses were not mentally confused. A widower whose wife could no longer recognize people and who was frequently covered in her own excrement said:

> 'I got frustrated at times. I couldn't do things I wanted to do. I got annoyed — gradually things dropped off. We used to go out to see friends but that got embarrassing, she'd use all the wrong cutlery. It got to the point where I was afraid she might do something terrible.'

In some of these cases an element of relief at the death was expressed. One woman who died of multiple sclerosis was described as mentally confused and depressed. She had been ill for twenty years and her husband had retired early to look after her:

> 'Friends and relatives would come in and see her sitting there in her chair, all clean and cheerful, she always had a smile for them, they didn't realize what I had to do to keep her like that. They'd say to her "How well you look today" and no-one would think to say how well I looked after her. I think the doctor and the nurse realized that I was on the edge of a breakdown myself. I wasn't getting proper sleep. I laid on the couch because I couldn't sleep with my wife. She kept calling all night, I never got no sleep.'

The widowed often seemed to accept the burden of caring that had been placed on them as their duty. Two widows said:

> 'It was like living in a vacuum really, it was all unreal, but I would not have had it any other way.'

> 'When you marry someone it is for life so it was my place to look after him.'

The feeling that they themselves, not only professionals, had done all they could, and that their husband or wife had been well looked after, may help reduce feelings of guilt after the death. As one widow said:

> 'The only thing that goes through my mind is "Did I do everything to help, did I do enough?" It keeps going through my mind.'

One widow continually referred to her feelings of guilt because she felt she had not given adequate care to her husband. Her husband was mentally confused and died of cancer. She said she did not pay him enough attention because she had not realized he was dying. She also said she had needed help to look after him, especially when he fell, but had not known whom to ask:

> 'He kept falling out of bed — the poor creature was on the floor. I couldn't help him. I was afraid to sleep. I went out for help but

everything was dark. I couldn't phone my daughter . . . my daughter said she wouldn't help me. They didn't understand how ill he was. . . . I was always thinking "Why is he always forgetting?" I didn't realize. One thing made me very upset. The doctor said he wasn't to have cigarettes so I took them away. I felt very sad about that, he could have had what he wanted (as he was dying).'

Almost a quarter of the widowed, 24%, said their spouse's ill-health had affected them financially. This proportion was higher for widows, 28%, than widowers, 18%. Although no differences were found with place of death or length of illness, deaths from cancer and bronchitis had more effects on finances than other deaths, 32% in comparison with 21%. It was pointed out earlier that cancer deaths also imposed the most restriction on the spouse's activities. Possibly more money had to be spent on special foods, clothing, or heating with these conditions and those dying of cancer were more likely to have been to hospital as outpatients in the last year than those dying from other causes, 68% compared with 40%. This may have led to some expense.

Those classified as working class were more likely to say they had been affected financially, 26%, than those classified as middle class, 15%. However, the widowed who said they were affected financially were also more likely to have had financial help, 57%, than those who said they were not affected, 35%. This still leaves 43% of those who said they were affected financially who received no financial help. Altogether, 23% received supplementary benefit before the death and 9% received a disability pension, 9% an attendance allowance, and 10% received help from a relative or other sources. One widow whose husband was chronically ill with bronchitis for twelve years and whom she nursed intensively for about six months was discouraged from claiming the attendance allowance by her general practitioner. She said the doctor told her:

'It wasn't worth it, he wouldn't be here long enough.'

We had no measure of whether the widowed would have qualified for an attendance allowance before the death so we cannot estimate the number who were eligible but who did not claim. However, as 26% had said their activities were severely restricted and 19% said they were fairly restricted because of the deceased's illness, probably

40 Life After A Death

more than the 9% receiving an attendance allowance were eligible for it. Those who were affected financially mentioned the cost of extra food, clothes, and heating as being the main problems:

> 'I had to keep getting him trousers, the others were falling off him. I had to get baby foods, Complan, and the nurse told me to get Ovaltine. The gas bill was high, we had to burn that night and day, same as the lights.'

It is clear that the care of dying people at home often imposes severe physical, financial, and psychological strains on their relatives. Wives and husbands generally take on this task willingly but often they do it unaided when appropriate help and support could mitigate the physical hardship, the social isolation, and the mental distress.

The role of the familiars

While the spouse bore the brunt of caring for the person who died, relatives and friends also helped in many instances. What was the extent of their involvement and how did it affect their lives? Interviews with the widowed person's familiars give some indication about this. Thirty per cent of the familiars said they had helped to care for the person who died[8] and just over half, 52%, said the person's illness had affected their life in some way.[9] Children of the widowed were more likely to say this than other familiars, 57% in comparison with 41%. Effects mentioned included emotional strain, the extra work involved in caring for the deceased and helping the couple, and disruptions to home life and work:

> 'At times they would send for me and I would have to have time off work.'

> 'Emotionally it upset me having to do and see what I did. I was on the verge of collapse. It was getting to the point where my husband was insisting that he [deceased] went into hospital.'

We also asked 'During the time —— was ill, was there anything you gave up or did less of?' Although 69% said there was nothing they had given up or done less of, 15% said they had given up something and

[8] Helping with dressing or undressing, getting in or out of bath, washing or shaving, being lifted at all, getting to the lavatory, help or care at night, anything else like that.
[9] 'Did ——'s illness/condition affect your life at all?'

Table 13   Things familiars have given up or done less of because of the illness

Activities:	%
Visiting friends or relatives	20
Going out to other social activities	22
Going on holiday	8
Entertaining people at home	13
Going to work	13
Other activities	4
Nothing	69
Number of familiars (= 100%)	211

16% had done less of something. The activities involved are shown above in *Table 13*. Giving up or cutting down on work activities is one of the things likely to have the most far-reaching effect on familiars' lives — especially financially. Children of the widowed were more likely to have cut down or given up work, 16% in comparison with 5% of other familiars.

Altogether, 7% of familiars regarded their activities before the death as 'severely restricted', 10% as 'fairly restricted', and 13% said they were 'a little restricted'. Sixty-nine per cent said they were 'not restricted' and one familiar gave another comment. Some of those who felt restricted added:

'Of course I didn't go anywhere.'

'We had to drop our normal way of living, and be in attendance all the time.'

'My whole life was revolving around my mother.'

Table 14 shows that familiars who were daughters of the widowed were more likely to have experienced restrictions, as were females generally. The existence of mental confusion in the deceased also had some impact on the familiars' activities.

Some examples of the effects of the illness on familiars' lives were:

'You could not go away from home for long, even shopping. You can't leave them if they are in one position, they need moving. If they get breathless they get distressed.'

'We [self and husband] were both definitely worn out and not only that — we went down with colds, which didn't help, and yet still had to fight on. Every third night over a period of a month we lost

Table 14   Restriction on the familiars' activities before the death

	Activities restricted	Number of familiars (= 100%)
Familiar's relationship to widowed:		
Daughter	42%	98
Son	22%	49
Other familiar	19%	64
Familiar's sex:		
Female	35%	144
Male	21%	67
Deceased mentally confused:		
Yes	39%	79
No	26%	129

sleep for a whole night with no chance of catching it up during the day-time. It was brain damage, you see, and he slept in the day and played us up all night. In the end he was trying to climb the walls but couldn't because his legs were bad. The nurses that came in just supervised . . . we had asked for a lot more help but they said they could only offer more help for terminal cases and cancers. . . . District nurses are only allocated to cancer patients and what Dad had [stroke] didn't qualify. We were cracking up. I was falling asleep and crying. But I felt I had to pull myself together because mother [widow] relied on me.'

'I had to practically re-organize my own life. As soon as I left home I had to go straight down and make breakfast and do the house-work, see to her [deceased], and things like that. I got the lunch and the shopping and then came back to anything that had to be done here. I went back again in the evening.'

'It was almost like not living. We all gave up communicating with each other. I had trouble with the children, I had trouble with my mother (the deceased) because I hit her. I got really angry one day because she just laughed when she made a mess of the bed. I just lashed out at her and hit her across the bottom. It was all trouble, trouble all the time.'

The last familiar, a daughter, had shared the nursing with the widower, who had had a stroke himself, and a district nurse, although the district nurse only started visiting during the last week of life. The deceased had gradually declined in health over a nine-month period after a stroke and was totally incontinent:

> 'She wasn't blessed with one big stroke to make that it. She got worse and worse – completely incontinent. The last weeks were unbelievable. If I wasn't a nursing auxiliary I couldn't have coped. I visited her every day. She had lived with me from May to August but in August she went into sheltered housing. I had to go there every day to look after her. The washing was endless. I quite shamelessly sneaked things into the hospital laundry [where works].'

She felt that insufficient help was given by the health and social services because everyone felt she knew enough about nursing to be able to cope – being a nursing auxiliary.

Other familiars also mentioned feeling irritable with the deceased during the illness:

> 'I used to get very irritable with her sometimes. You'd say something and she just couldn't take it. She mumbled a lot and was cross if you couldn't understand. She changed a lot after the first stroke. She'd never been one to say anything nasty about people but she went quite different, always finding fault and being bitter. It used to get on my nerves.'

These quotations show that disruption to the lives of some of the familiars had been extensive. So, although relatively few were severely restricted, if such people could be identified and their problems alleviated the relief would be considerable; it is not a question of large amounts of resources but of appropriate distribution.

The death

Almost half, 45%, the widowed had been in the same room as their spouse when they died. This was made up of a quarter who were on their own, and a fifth who also had relatives or friends with them. In a further 6% of deaths, other relatives or friends but not the spouse were with the deceased at the time of death. So almost half, 49%, died with no relatives or friends with them. As expected, those who died in a hospital, or other institution, were more likely to die alone, 74%, than those who died at home, 15%. These are similar to the proportions found by Cartwright, Hockey, and Anderson (1973).

Even when the widowed stayed overnight at the hospital to be with their spouses, they were often absent at the time of death:

'I was at the hospital all Friday night, and I was just going to leave here [home] to visit him again when his nephews came round. They were going to visit him at 9 o'clock. Then I had a 'phone call to say he passed away.'

'Although I had been there (in hospital) for eight or nine days, I hardly left his side. The day he died I'd had the opportunity to come home for a couple of hours as I was feeling the strain, and two hours after I left he died.'

We asked the widowed who were not present at the death whether they would have preferred to have been with their spouses then. Over half, 59%, said they would. Being with the person at the time of death to say 'goodbye' may affect the immediate adjustment to, and acceptance of, the death; feelings of guilt or anxiety may be lessened:

'I always look back and say "I wish I could have said so and so, or done this or that". The last time I saw him he had a mask over his face.'

'Yes, I'd like to have been with him − seen the last of the poor old soul − especially as they said he was sensible at the end.'

'I'd like to know what happened − a chance to say "Bye bye" and "Thanks for what you've done". I'd like to know if he called out or suffered before he went.'

'[I'd lost the last] chance I had to see my husband. This is why I can't sleep. I don't know if he went in agony − if he asked for me − I know nothing. I never saw him at all. I couldn't get to the hospital in all that snow − I had no car, nothing. I never saw him again. I think its disgusting. We've never asked anyone for anything yet they [hospital] couldn't help us at the end − couldn't they have once sent out an ambulance? I feel very bitter.'

'I think I would have liked to have said a few things to him, to thank him for all the good years we had and to reassure him that I'd be able to manage without him. I would really have liked to go at the same time because when you're as close as we were you feel like that.'

'He died in the ambulance. They've stopped people going in the ambulance now I believe because of the difficulty of them getting back home. That hurt me. I would have liked to have been with him.'

Over half of those who were not present at the death, 60%, had seen the body afterwards. This often seemed to give some comfort to the widowed:

'They'd done just as I asked them at the hospital. They crossed his hands and put a crucifix between them. It was always his wish to be buried with that crucifix.'

However, only 16% of those who had not seen the body would have preferred to have done so. These widows and widowers had generally chosen not to see the body:

'No, I was asked if I wanted to but I want to remember her as she lived.'

'I am glad I can remember him as I last saw him − jolly and waving.'

When the husband or wife had died at home a doctor had usually either been there or had come to see them after they died; but 14% of the widowed said no doctor had come. Three would have liked one to do so. One widow told us:

'The doctor said "If he dies in the middle of the night don't send for me if it's after 11 pm at night, just come to the surgery and I'll give you a death certificate". I think that's awful don't you? That's just what did happen too and it haunts me at night thinking about it. What if the undertaker took him and he wasn't dead?'

Others said they did not mind.

Immediately after the death

Most of the widowed, three-quarters, felt they had known enough about what to do when someone died. But 12% felt it would have been helpful if they had known more and 12% gave other answers. Some of the things they wanted to know more about were:

'What to do shortly after the death occurs − the immediate things.'

'The physical side of things. I know about legal matters.'

'I didn't know anything − who to contact or anything.'

Most of those who felt they knew enough did so because of previous experience, but 13% said someone had told them. Relatives had helped most of these; only one had been given information by a general practitioner. There is a definite gap in information services here – affecting between one in eight and one in four of the elderly widowed. When the spouse had died at home the widowed were more likely to say it would have been helpful if they had known more about what to do – 18% of them said this compared with 8% of those whose spouse had died in hospital. This suggests that general practitioners could help with this, but as we will see later they are only in contact with a minority of the widowed at this point. As long as this is so they will not be able either to advise about this themselves or to direct people to an appropriate source.

Summary

Few people married to men of 65 or more or women aged 60 or more are plunged into widowhood without warning. For most, widowhood is preceded by a lengthy period of illness: a quarter of the husbands and wives who died had been ill for as long as ten years and for two-thirds it was at least a year. And for most of their illness they were looked after at home. Although half the deaths took place in a hospital or institution, only one in twelve of the married people who died spent as long as three months of the last year of their lives in hospital. So the majority were ill for some time at home and while there many needed care with such personal things as dressing, washing, or getting to the lavatory. Wives and husbands bore the brunt of this care for three-quarters of those who needed it. Two-thirds of the prospective widows and widowers led restricted lives during this period and for some the restrictions were severe, particularly when the spouse they were caring for was mentally confused.

A fifth of the widowed felt that more help was needed in caring for the personal needs of the person who died, and a few were directly critical of the professional care in hospital or from the general practitioner.

Quotations from interviews with the widowed and from those with their familiars reveal some of the hardships, the anguish, the stresses, and the strains involved in caring for dying people at home. Most of the wives and husbands accepted this task willingly but for some the burden was too great, and a number lacked recognition from relatives and friends and adequate support from professionals. Extracts from two of the more poignant quotations were:

'No-one would think to say how well I looked after her.'

'I was coping allright so they [doctors] didn't come. It was 24-hour constant attendance for me.'

3 Information and discussion about the death

In the previous chapter we saw that a number of the widowed talked about the information and the lack of information they had from their general practitioners when they were describing the doctors' care of their spouse. How much did the prospective widows and widowers know about the prognosis of their spouse's illness? How much did they want to know? How many of the people who were dying realized this? What part did the general practitioners play in this; and how did they view their role? These are the questions raised in this chapter.

Awareness of the widows and widowers[1]

The widowed were asked whether they were able to find out all they wanted to know about their spouse's illness and what the effects were likely to be. Almost a third, 32%, said they were not, and a further 7% would have liked something explained to them in more detail. Some of the widowed who would have liked to know more felt the medical and nursing staff were reluctant to discuss the illness:

'They wouldn't answer your questions so you never got anywhere.'

'I tried to talk to the doctor but he didn't seem to want to talk.'

'They tell plenty of white lies in hospital.'

[1] Those 9% whose spouse died instantaneously or who were ill for less than a week have been excluded from this discussion, and from the next section about the dying person's awareness.

Lack of communication on the part of professionals rather than dispelling fears may actually raise and reinforce anxieties and frustrations. Awareness can be raised and anxieties created by overheard conversations, bodily symptoms, changes in treatment routines, and in others' behaviour, and even by refusals by professionals to give direct answers to questions. Some comments illustrate this:

'It was a problem, they kept putting you off. You couldn't get a straight answer. All you got was "It'll take time".'

'I was never told he was suspected of having his complaint. [Cancer.] I had no idea, perhaps they thought I couldn't take it. I got worried when I saw the flesh going off his arms.'

When asked about the type of professionals they had spoken to about the illness, most of the widowed, 60% of them, said they had spoken to a general practitioner, 39% to another doctor. A third had spoken to a nurse and a quarter to a vicar, priest, or rabbi. One in four had not spoken to a professional at all.

Although almost a third had not been able to find out all they wanted to know, only 10% said they would have liked to have talked, or talked more, about the illness and what was likely to happen, and 2% were uncertain about this. The majority, nine out of ten, of the small proportion who said they would have liked more or at least some discussion, would have preferred to talk to a professional, and most of these mentioned a doctor. The apparent contradictory attitudes among those who said they had not been able to find out all they wanted to know, but did not want to talk about it more, reflect people's uncertainties and fears over communication about terminal illnesses — many may have a desire for knowledge but are still afraid to possess it. One widow commented:

'I often felt like it [asking] but I dare not.'

Wishing that some things could have been done differently was clearly related to their satisfaction with the information they had been given about their spouse's illness. Among those who were able to find out all they wanted to know in as much detail as they wanted, only 17% would have liked something done differently. This proportion rose to 26% of those wanting more detailed information and to 34% of those who said they had not been able to find out what they wanted to know.

Three-fifths, 61%, said they had spoken to relatives about the illness and what was likely to happen, and three out of ten, 30%, spoke to friends and neighbours. Amongst non-professionals also, the widowed recognized a tendency to shield them from any knowledge which may have been upsetting:

'I couldn't find out anything. They never told me nothing, but my son, who's a nurse, found out and explained things to me. But he didn't tell me she had cancer and was going to die.'

'I would like to have known but my son didn't tell me. He thought it was best for me not to know. He thought I had enough to put up with, but I would have liked to have known.'

Others tended to deny the truth to themselves:

'A lot of the neighbours used to see how ill she was getting and they used to comment. But you yourself don't want to see the truth before you.'

We asked the widowed whether they would say they knew, half knew, or did not know at all that their spouse was likely to die soon and how they felt about this. Almost half, 43%, said they had known, almost a fifth, 17%, half knew, and 40% did not know. Cartwright, Hockey, and Anderson (1973) found a higher level of awareness among the widowed they interviewed: 60% of the wives and husbands of people aged 65 or more said they knew their spouse was unlikely to recover, 12% half knew, 28% did not know.[2] The comparison suggests that the widowed had been less aware of the probable outcome on the more recent survey − a rather surprising finding, particularly as we will see that among general practitioners over the same period there seemed to have been a trend to more open communication.

We asked the widowed how they felt about the amount of knowledge of the condition and prognosis they had had, that is whether the situation was best as it was or whether they would have liked to have known more or less, as the case may be. The proportions saying the situation was best as it was declined with decreasing knowledge. Among those who knew their spouse was likely to die soon, the majority,

[2] The questions on the two surveys were slightly different, the earlier one asking whether they knew, or half knew, their spouse was 'unlikely to recover', and the current one if they knew or half knew he or she was 'likely to die soon'. Previously published results cover deaths of all ages.

94%, said that this was best as it was and it would not have been better if they had not known:

'It prepared me for it, and it didn't come as so much of a shock.'

'If you realize I think you can give more help and take more strain off them willingly. You don't get the sudden shocks.'

Slightly fewer of those who half knew, 87%, said this was best as it was − no more or less knowledge would have been preferred.

Those who did not know tended to be less accepting of the situation: just over two-thirds, 67%, said this was best as it was, while almost a quarter, 23%, said it would have been better if they had known. The widowed who did not know but felt the situation was best as it was tended to say the knowledge would have been too much of a strain for them:

'I couldn't have stood up to it. You see what I'm going through now.'

'If you know too much you worry yourself.'

The 23% who would have liked to have known mostly felt that the death might have been less of a shock and that they would have behaved differently towards the deceased. This period of widowhood (that is, at the time of the interview − around five months after the death) often seemed to be a time of reflecting on instances of neglect or unkindness:

'If I'd known I wouldn't have pushed him around so much.'

'I was stunned. I couldn't believe that he had gone. I couldn't get it through to me. It would have made it easier [if I'd known] to speak to him and do things for him without hurting him.'

Further evidence that a substantial proportion of the widowed who had not known their spouse was terminally ill would have liked more information about the illness and prognosis comes from the data in *Table 15*. The proportion who said they had been unable to find out all they wanted to know about their spouse's illness and how it was likely to affect him or her, rose from just under a quarter of those who had realized their spouse was dying to just over two-fifths of those who had not known. In addition more of those who did not know or were doubtful about the prognosis said they would have liked something to have been done differently. This too is shown in *Table 15*.

Table 15   The widowed's knowledge of prognosis, their ability to find out all they wanted to know, and wishes about things being done differently

	Widowed's knowledge of prognosis			All widowed
	Knew	*Half knew*	*Did not know*	
Knowledge:	%	%	%	%
Unable to find out all wanted to know	23	30	42	32
Able to find out things but would have liked more detail	7	13	6	7
Able to find out and did not want more detail	69	57	50	60
Other comment	1	–	2	1
Wished something had been done differently:	17%	23%	31%	23%
Number of widowed (=100%)	136	56	120	317

The widowed who knew or half knew were more likely to have talked to professionals about the illness and what was likely to happen – 83% in comparison with 63% of those who did not know. They were also more likely to have talked to relatives or friends, 78%, than those who did not know, 54%.

Those in Social Class V were less likely to know the prognosis, 26%, than those in other social classes, 45%. As no differences were found with social class and talking about the condition, it is possible that the relationship with social class and knowledge of the prognosis may be explained by the less adequate information that people in lower social classes receive from their doctors (Cartwright 1979). Although a relationship was found between knowledge of the prognosis and talking about the condition, still a significant minority, 29%, remained who had spoken to a general practitioner but who were not aware of the prognosis. Some professionals may not have been definite about the prognosis themselves, others may have decided to withhold the information, while some of the potential widows and widowers may not have taken in or accepted the information they were given.

Table 16   Widowed's knowledge of prognosis by cause of death

	Cause of death							
	Malignant neoplasm	*Ischaemic heart disease*	*Cerebrovascular accidents*	*Other circulatory diseases*	*Pneumonia and influenza*	*Bronchitis*	*Other*	*All causes*
Widowed's knowledge:	%	%	%	%	%	%	%	%
Knew	60	35	40	34	35	40	45	43
Half knew	19	18	30	8	9	20	14	17
Did not know	21	47	30	58	56	40	41	40
Number of deaths (= 100%)	81	95	33	26	32	25	29	321

The widowed were more likely to have known the prognosis if the cause of death was cancer, as *Table 16* shows, probably because the illness may be more visible in these cases:

'They all knew. You could see it in him. He had gone down a lot after radium. The flesh just dropped off him.'

The finding that respondents who said they wished things had gone differently before the death were less likely to have known the prognosis than those who said there was nothing they would have liked done differently, 31% in comparison with 47%, suggests that knowledge of the imminence of death may enable husbands and wives to prepare themselves better. Some comments about this were:

'I only wish they'd have told me. If I'd known she'd had cancer we would have spoken and I would have liked to have talked to her about it. But I didn't know.'

'If I'd known I'd have done more for him.'

'If we'd known he was going to die we'd rather have had him at home.'

'Only that we'd spoken a bit more before he'd died. I would have liked to have been prepared.'

Better preparation, resulting from knowledge, may also lead to fewer guilt feelings after the death.

The dying person's awareness

We asked the widowed whether they thought their husband or wife knew, or half knew, or did not know at all, that he or she was likely to die soon, and how they themselves felt about this. Almost half, 44%, said they thought he or she had known, 14% said they thought the person had half known, and 30% were said not to have known. In 12% of cases the respondent was uncertain. When these findings are compared with those of Cartwright, Hockey, and Anderson (1973), it would seem that there has been a change in the opposite direction to the one for the widowed themselves. The proportion of people who died who were thought to have known that they were unlikely to recover had increased from 37% in 1969 to 44% in 1979, while the proportion who did not know fell from 43% to 30%.

On the more recent study a similar proportion of the widowed as deceased spouses knew about the prognosis. And, as *Table 17* shows, their knowledge, or lack of it, was clearly related. However, in a significant minority of instances, 15%, the widowed did not know but in retrospect thought the deceased had realized it or half knew, while in 13% the widowed had known but thought their husband or wife did not or only half knew.

Table 17   The widowed's and the deceased's knowledge of prognosis

	Widowed's own knowledge		
	Knew	*Half knew*	*Did not know*
Widowed's estimate of deceased's knowledge:	%	%	%
Knew	62	41	26
Half knew	12	29	11
Did not know	17	18	48
Uncertain	9	12	15
Number of widowed (= 100%)	138	56	126

In this last group will be some who illustrate Glaser and Strauss's (1965) category of suspected awareness in which the patient was suspicious of the diagnosis but not sure, and others for whom there was a mutual pretence, the patient and family both knowing but denying knowledge to each other. In both instances they cannot easily talk to each other because of the 'conspiracy of silence' surrounding them. Patients may pick up signals about the likely death because of the reluctance of family and staff to initiate discussions about it.

We asked the widowed whether they felt the deceased's state of awareness was best as it was, or whether it would have been better if the deceased had known more or less, depending on the case. The majority, 83%, of those who said the deceased knew said this was best as it was, as did 95% of those who said the deceased half knew, and 80% of those who said the deceased did not know. It may be too disturbing for the widowed to admit that a different situation might have been better:

> 'What would be the point of lying to her? The doctor didn't try to bluff her at all. She wanted to prepare herself and she did. She was ready. She was totally aware — she chose the hymns for her funeral.'

> 'I don't think he would have fought his way back to life as he did these last eighteen months if he'd known for sure it was cancer. He wouldn't have bothered any more.'

Analysis by whether the widows or widowers wished anything had been done differently showed that those who had not realized their spouse was dying but in retrospect thought that their husband or wife knew or half realized this were the ones most likely to wish something had been done differently: 33% of them felt this; whereas only 8% of those who knew themselves but thought their spouse had not known would have liked things to have been different, and 22% of the intermediate group. It appears that even those who preferred to face the truth themselves did not all feel that it was appropriate for the dying person to do so. But of course the views of the people who died may have been very different. Hinton (1980) talked to eighty married people with fatal neoplastic disease and found that two-thirds recognized that they might or would die soon. He concluded that many patients with cancer would like greater opportunity to discuss their situation more fully but not necessarily with the doctor. In another study Jones (1981) concluded that a policy of telling all patients or of telling none was unlikely to suit more than half.

Although there was no relationship with length of illness and the widowed's knowledge of the prognosis, the deceased was less likely to be said to have known the prognosis if he or she was ill for less than three months, 28% in comparison with 46% of those who were ill for longer than this.

Those dying from bronchitis were the ones thought to have been most likely to have been aware that they were likely to die soon. Apart from that, those dying of cancer were no less likely to have known their prognosis than those dying from other diseases. (The figures are in *Table 18*.) This is different from Duff and Hollingshead's (1968) finding that in three-quarters of the deaths studied, where doctors avoided telling patients their diagnosis, the disease category was cancer. On the other hand, in our study, cancer deaths stood out in that for them more of the widowed than of the deceased had known the prognosis. For cancer deaths, then, it appears that communication of the diagnosis was made to the spouse rather than to the deceased, and that there is some attempt to protect the patient from knowledge of the prognosis. This emerged more clearly in the study by Cartwright, Hockey, and Anderson (1973) where it was found that people dying from cancer were also thought less likely to have known what was wrong with them than people dying of other diseases.

Although no relationship was found between sex and the widowed person's knowledge, women who died were thought more likely not to know the prognosis, 37%, than men, 26%. Perhaps people are more likely to raise the subject of the outcome with men who die, under the assumption that they may have financial or business affairs to make arrangements about. But no relationship with social class and the deceased's (unlike the widowed person's) knowledge was found.

Who, if anyone, had talked to the person who died about what was likely to happen? Only 3% of those who were thought to have known they were dying were said by the widows or widowers to have talked to a doctor about this, and only 2% to another type of professional. More, 19%, had spoken to their husband or wife and 7% to relatives. Altogether 25% of those who knew had talked to someone about it, while the majority were thought to have realized it without discussing it with anyone.

In contrast to knowledge about the prognosis, a significant trend was found with communication with the deceased and social class.

Table 18   Deceased's knowledge of prognosis by cause of death

	Cause of death							
	Malignant neoplasm	*Ischaemic heart disease*	*Cerebrovascular accidents*	*Other circulatory diseases*	*Pneumonia and influenza*	*Bronchitis*	*Other*	*All causes*
Deceased's knowledge:	%	%	%	%	%	%	%	%
Knew	46	46	28	48	33	64	41	44
Half knew	17	12	18	16	25	8	3	14
Did not know	25	33	36	20	33	12	45	30
Uncertain if knew	12	9	18	16	9	16	10	12
Number of deaths (= 100%)	81	95	33	25	33	25	29	321

The proportion who said no-one had spoken to the deceased about what was likely to happen increased from 62% in Social Classes I and II to 90% in Social Class V.

We asked the widowed whether, looking back, they would have liked to have talked, or talked more, to their spouses about what was likely to happen. Almost a fifth, 19%, said they would:

'Yes, in a way, because I would have liked to have said "Goodbye" to him.'

'I would have liked to, I've said things to him that I wouldn't have said if I had known.'

The role of the general practitioner

The general practitioner appeared to play a key role in talking to the husband or wife about their spouse's illness and possible death. He or she was the professional person the widowed were most likely to have talked to. Three-fifths of the widowed whose spouse had been ill for

Table 19   Widows' and widowers' views of general practitioner by whether they had discussed their spouse's illness or possible death with their doctor

	Proportion who had discussed this with general practitioner	Number of widowed (= 100%)
Finds general practitioner:		
Very sympathetic	68%	132
Fairly sympathetic	53%	45
Rather unsympathetic	43%	21
Easy to talk to	64%	272
Not easy to talk to	43%	37
Thinks doctor has time to discuss things:		
Yes	66%	241
No	40%	62
Regards relationship with general practitioner as:		
Friendly	68%	133
Businesslike	55%	168
Felt general practitioner's care of spouse was:		
Very good	65%	197
Fairly good	58%	72
Not very good	39%	28

a week or more before they died, said they had talked to a general practitioner about the illness and what was likely to happen. This proportion fell from 75% of the widowed who said they knew that their spouse was likely to die soon, to 57% of those who said they 'half knew', and 44% of those who had not known. Looking at this the other way, of those who had talked to a general practitioner about their husband's or wife's illness, just over half, 54%, said they knew he or she was likely to die, 17% 'half knew', and 29% did not know. The majority of those who had talked to a general practitioner, 70%, said they were able to find out all they wanted to know and did not want anything explained in more detail, but 22% had felt they could not get all the information they wanted, and a further 8% would have liked more explanation.

Those who had talked to a general practitioner about their husband's or wife's illness and impending or possible death seemed to have a better relationship with their doctor in a number of ways. This is shown in *Table 19*. Of course it is not possible to tell whether they found the doctor sympathetic because he or she had talked about their husband's or wife's illness, or whether they were able to talk about the illness because they found the doctor sympathetic. Almost certainly it goes both ways. But either way, the widowed person's feelings about the doctor's sympathy and care of their spouse is related to discussion about illness and death.

The proportion of the widowed who had discussed their spouse's illness with a general practitioner was the same if the person died at home or in hospital. And it did not vary significantly with social class. Sixty-six per cent of widowers said they had discussed the illness with a general practitioner compared with 56% of widows, but this difference might have occurred by chance. Those who had discussed it with relatives or friends were also more likely to have talked to a general practitioner about it: 68% of them had done so compared with 43% of those who had not talked to relatives or friends about it. We do not know which happened first or who initiated the discussions, but it seems that discussion with a friend or relative may stimulate or lead to discussion with a general practitioner and vice versa. Some people, 15%, had talked to other professional people but not a general practitioner. The situation is summarized in *Table 20*.

The proportion of the widowed who said they felt they would have liked to have talked, or to have talked more, about what was likely to

Table 20   Impending widows' or widowers' discussion of spouse's illness and possible death with different types of people

Discussed with:	%
General practitioner and friends or relatives	46
General practitioner but not friends or relatives	14
Relatives and friends but not general practitioner	22
Neither general practitioner nor relatives or friends but some professional person	5
No-one	13
Number of widowed * (= 100%)	322

* Excludes 32 whose spouse died instantaneously with no previous illness, or within a week of becoming ill, and 7 for whom inadequate information was obtained.

happen was 19%. This was similar for those who had talked to a general practitioner, and for those who had not. This lack of difference presumably arises because of a number of variations which work in different ways. If general practitioners are more likely to discuss this with relatives who want to do so, the discussion may not always meet all their needs and may sometimes stimulate a desire to talk about things more.

General practitioners had talked to many of the future widows and widowers about their spouse's illness and death, but it seemed that few had talked to the person who was dying. As we showed earlier, only 3% of those who were thought to have known they were dying were said to have talked to a doctor about this. And if we consider the whole group, although over half were thought to have had some inkling of the situation, few had talked to anyone about it; 85% of the widowed said neither they nor anyone else had talked to their spouse about what was likely to happen. Two per cent were said to have talked to a doctor about it; more, 12%, had talked to their husband or wife.

This experience of the widowed, that general practitioners are willing to talk to the surviving spouse but not to the dying person, ties up with some aspects of the general practitioners' views of their role.

General practitioners' views of their role in discussion of impending death

Doctors were asked whether, if open communication about the future is made possible between the dying patient and their spouse, they thought the widowed person's reasonable adaptation to bereavement was enhanced, and the dying person was likely to accept the situation more calmly. Nearly three-quarters, 74%, thought the spouse's adaptation was enhanced; three-fifths, 60%, that the dying patient accepted his or her situation more calmly. (Nearly half, 47%, agreed to both propositions, 7% to neither, and 5% made other comments.) But while recognizing the advantages of open communication there were situations in which they felt it inappropriate for them to take the initiative in moving towards it. In our questionnaire we stated that whether a person should be told that they were dying probably depended on a number of different things, but asked the doctors what they would probably do in three situations, each relating to an elderly married person with a terminal illness who would almost certainly die within six weeks. In one situation the patient asks: 'This won't kill me doctor will it?'. The most common reply, by 39% of doctors, was that they would agree and a further 20% said they would pass it off as a joke. However 25% said they would tell the patient the truth and 16% made other comments. Some of these last were:

'I usually let this lead to a discussion on death and dying to explore the patient's and the relatives' attitudes before dealing with the specific question.'

'I would suggest that the illness is serious and the situation a bit worrying.'

'Be non-committal, never lie but never pass it off as a joke.'

'Try to discuss their knowledge of the illness and what they want to know.'

Many of those who said they would tell the patient the truth qualified this with such phrases as 'gradually', 'gently', 'indirectly', and 'but never with finality'.

A rather similar question was asked in a study carried out ten years previously in 1969 (Cartwright, Hockey, and Anderson 1973). In that study fewer general practitioners, 13%, said they would tell the patient the truth, and more that they would 'pass it off as a joke or change the subject' − 34%.

The second situation related to a patient who asked directly 'Is this going to kill me doctor?'. Over this there was greater consensus, with 61% reporting that they would say 'yes probably'; 22% would say they did not know, 6% would say no, 5% would change the subject, and 6% gave other answers. The question asked in the earlier study was not strictly comparable as it referred to 'a businessman of 55', but similar proportions in both 1969 and 1979 said they would tell the person the truth or change the subject, while fewer in 1979 would say no − 6% against 12% in the earlier study − and more would say they did not know − 22% in 1979, 10% in 1969.

In relation to a patient who did not raise the topic and seemed unaware of the prognosis, 91% in 1979 said they would tell the spouse only, 4% would tell the spouse and the patient, 1% would not tell either, and 4% made other comments. These are similar responses to those in 1969, but again the questions are not entirely comparable since the earlier one related to 'a mother of 35 with young children'.

On balance there seems a slight trend towards more open communication: in one example towards telling the patient the truth, in another away from denial of the truth. The size of the change is much smaller than that reported by Novack, *et al.* (1979) who in 1977 found that 98% of physicians said that their usual policy was to tell cancer patients the truth, in contrast to 1961 when 12% adopted that policy. They also asked about the bases for the policies and conclude: 'Clinical experience was the determining factor in shaping two opposite policies. Physicians are still basing their policies on emotion-laden personal convictions rather than the outcome of properly designed scientific studies.'

While there was considerable difference of opinion between the doctors about what patients should be told, there was fairly general agreement that if patients were to be told that they were unlikely to recover then the general practitioner was usually the best person to do this: 82% of doctors thought this, 16% thought the patient's husband or wife, 10% a vicar, priest, or minister. (Some mentioned more than one person.) There was also fairly general agreement that a spouse should generally be informed when an elderly person was dying; over a third of the doctors, 35%, thought there were no exceptions to this, most of the others mentioning certain mental or physical conditions in which they felt it would not be appropriate:

'Too emotionally unstable or equally seriously ill.'

A small minority, 3%, said this should not be done if the patient did not want his or her spouse to be informed.

Discussion

Obviously doctors find it hard to achieve what they see as the ideal situation in practice. Most feel open communication is a good thing, but while general practitioners feel they are the most appropriate people to talk to dying patients about their impending death, the evidence of the widowed suggests that they do so with few patients. They are much more likely to be involved in discussions with impending widows or widowers and these discussions are appreciated and seem to create or enhance a sympathetic and understanding relationship with the widowed.

What is inevitably missing from our study is the viewpoint of the people who died: we do not know how they would have felt about a situation in which their condition and prognosis was more often discussed with their spouse than with them. To us it seems that once a person has been diagnosed as having a terminal illness there is a danger that some doctors cease to regard such a patient as a person with rights and feelings. Few doctors, 3%, voiced the opinion that the dying person's wishes should be taken into consideration when deciding whether or not to inform a spouse about the prognosis. And we wonder about the ethics of giving such information so often to the spouse and so rarely to the patient. A study by Jones (1981) suggests that about half the patients with a terminal illness want to know this. A consecutive series of patients with an inoperable cancer were told that after investigation they would be given a firm diagnosis if they cared to ask, but that if they did not care for medical details there would be no need to ask. Forty-nine per cent asked for the diagnosis. This contrasts with 1% of the dying people in this study who were thought to have known they were dying and discussed this with a doctor. Kübler-Ross (1970) has said that doctors should listen for cues from patients which enable them to elicit their willingness to face the reality. This takes time, experience, and sensitivity, but we feel it is important to do this before informing the spouse while leaving the patient in ignorance or doubt. Patients may become anxious when faced with uncertainty; and they may lose trust in, and respect for, a doctor they suspect of lying.

4 Practical needs and circumstances in the early months of widowhood

What practical problems do men and women face after the death of their spouses? What proportion are left living alone and how many move or consider moving? Just how many alternatives are open to them? This chapter looks at these issues, together with the domestic and financial situations of the widowed, and the impact of sudden role changes.

Those who moved

Few people in the present sample had moved by the time we saw them: 11 widows and 6 widowers, 5%. Tunstall (1966) also found that older widows were unlikely to move. In our study, five of the widowed had moved within a month of their spouse's death, the majority waited longer, and most of the moves were fairly local, 12 out of the 17 moving less than five miles. Nine still lived alone while 8 had moved in with their sons or daughters and their families. Why did these widows and widowers move?

Four did so because their homes were too big for them now and were regarded as unmanageable and expensive. One of these, a widow who moved in with her daughter and son-in-law, said:

'Because I was in rather a large house with rather a large garden and no-one to help, and my daughter said "Come and live with us". I had a bad back and a bad leg. . . . I would have liked to have kept my own home but I am very comfortable so I won't grumble.'

Five had planned the move before their spouse died: one of these couples planned to live nearer their son and had bought a house near him; in the remaining four the moves were for the benefit of the spouse who had died:

> 'I moved for my husband's sake. We were to get the flat beforehand. I asked for the flat for my husband because I was afraid of him falling up and down the stairs. . . . I like it but I regret he isn't with me. I was looking forward to the two of us going into it.'

> 'We had the health visitor visit us. It was an old terraced house. She said the wife would have been better off (if we moved). . . . She had to have a wheelchair. We had no hot and cold running water. . . . There was no bath . . . and it was a cold house. We were going to move just two days after she died.'

Three moved because their families had persuaded them to:

> 'I've got the one daughter . . . and she's not happy if she can't see me. She works too, she has three boys and it's all so expensive, she couldn't come to see me much. . . . I had to give in as I knew she would worry.'

> 'My daughter wouldn't let me stop there on my own − it was cold there.'

One other widow was forced to move as her home had been tied to her husband's work − he had been a market gardener. The house and garden were sold together after his death. This widow was facing a number of problems − her son had died a fortnight before the death of her husband and she was still caring for her other son who was epileptic. Finally, four said they felt a need to get away, one of these had also recently lost a close friend:

> 'I simply broke up with my nerves. I couldn't settle in that house. There were too many memories.'

> 'I couldn't have stopped there. My neighbour died five days after my husband. We had been friends for forty-two years. We were proper fools together. If she wanted me she knocked on the wall. Her husband had been dead for fourteen years. I couldn't have stopped there without her.'

How stressful was the move to a new home? Loss of a home has been compared to other forms of bereavement (Hooper and Ineichen 1979), and moving to a new neighbourhood may be bewildering, disorienting, and lonely. Glick, Weiss, and Parkes (1974) found that widows who move after a death tend to regret it. All those in the present study, however, said they were glad they had moved when they did. They all regarded their new homes as very convenient for them. Also, when asked an open question concerning their feelings about their homes, four-fifths made positive or neutral comments in comparison with two-thirds of those who had not moved. On the other hand, a third of those who had moved said they were sorry to have left the memories associated with their last home behind, and two of those who had planned the move with their spouses expressed regret that they were not able to move together. One widower wondered about the wisdom of the move:

'I still wonder if it was wise to move here. There are always times when you think you may have made a mistake.'

This widower, together with four others, still felt unsettled and felt they might move again. One, who had once lived in Australia, thought he might go back there; the one who felt the move might have been a mistake said he might re-marry — he said he had already had two offers; a widow who lived with her daughter and her family, said she might not always be able to manage the stairs; and, finally, one widow was worried about becoming a burden on her daughter and the family she lived with.

We found on our follow-up of the pilot sample one year after the first interview, that few of the widowed had moved during that period. And Hooper and Ineichen (1979) found that, despite the existence of stress resulting from an unsatisfactory move, stressed families are unlikely to move again.

We asked the widowed who had moved in with others whether there was anything they had to do or could not do because of sharing a home. No problems were reported and all said they got on well with the people they shared with. On the other hand, of the nine who moved into a home alone, two had found living alone fairly difficult to accept and three had found it very difficult:

'I don't like it — nobody to talk to or discuss things with.'

'I get depressed now. I'm lost now because I've nothing to do.'

'I get some nights that I say to myself "What do I go to bed for? It's not worth it". I read something to fill in my time. I feel empty, nothing to rush for.'

How did other widows and widowers feel about sharing their home or living alone?

The home sharers

Twenty-two per cent of the widowed lived with others. The people they lived with were usually sons and daughters. Seventeen per cent of all the widowed shared with their children. The household composition of all the widowed is shown in *Table 21*. Apart from the 78% who lived alone, 14% shared with one other person, and 8% were in larger households of three to five people. The majority of those living with children, seven-tenths, shared their home with single children who had never married; one in seven lived with married children and a tenth with children whose marriage had broken up through divorce, separation, or widowhood. (A few lived with children in more than one category.)

Table 21   Type of household

Household composition:	%
Lives alone	78
Lives with	
1 child only	9
2 or more children only	3
Child(ren) + others	5
1 sibling or sibling-in-law only	3
Unrelated people only	1
Other combinations	1
Number of widowed (= 100%)	361

There was no difference between the widows and widowers in the proportion living alone, but the older widowed aged 65 or more were, if anything, more likely to be living on their own: 80% of them did so compared with 68% of the younger widowed. This is probably because the younger ones are more likely to have children who have not yet married. Only 20% of the widowed who had any single children lived alone compared with 90% of others. There was no difference in the proportions living on their own between those who had no children and those who only had children who were or had been married.

How did the widowed feel about sharing a home? When asked,

95% of those sharing a home said they got on with the other people there 'very well', and 4% said 'fairly well'. One widow said 'not very well'. This widow's brother had moved in with her after the death of his brother-in-law. He had recently returned from Australia and was staying temporarily with the widow. She commented:

> 'We haven't got the same temperaments. I'm quick-tempered. My husband got adjusted to me with my temperament. Everyone's got different ways haven't they? I'd rather be on my own.'

A few said there were things they either could not do, 4%, or had to do, 8%, because of sharing a home:

> 'You like to sit and wash your feet − or something like that − I like to sit and be nice and quiet and have a cup of tea on my own. I like a bit of privacy. There's things you can do with a husband that you can take for granted, it's only natural, but when you've got somebody else in the house you just can't do the same.'

> 'I have to have the TV on when I'd rather read.'

> 'I've got to get the meals for the lad [son]. The lad likes me here − I call him a lad but he's fifty-one. I could go and stay with my daughter − but I can't because of my son. I can't just lock up and go.'

While some of the widowed home sharers were essentially looking after unmarried children, others were being cared for by children who were married and had their own families. The effect on their lives is discussed in a later chapter, but some comments of those who were living with the widowed illustrate the type of problems faced:

> 'She gets fed up with (doing) all the clearing up that I don't get round to doing.'

> 'She wants to be here but I think she's worried because I can't go to work and I'm losing money.'

> 'She moans a bit at times because I do things my way. I take an even longer time to do things when she gets on at me.'

Apart from the home sharers being more likely to have unmarried children, were there any other differences between the widowed who lived with others and those who lived alone? Shanas, *et al.* (1968) found that among elderly people those living with children tended to be older, in poorer health, and with a lower income than others.

Fewer differences between the home sharers and those living alone were found in this study. There were no differences in terms of reported financial problems or health but, if anything, more working-class than middle-class widows and widowers lived with others. The proportions were 24% and 16% respectively, a difference which did not quite reach the level of statistical significance.

Living alone

What of the majority of the widowed, 78%, who were now living alone, often for the first time in their lives? When asked how they felt about this[1] 48% made negative comments such as they were nervous, lonely, or isolated. Twenty-nine per cent made neutral comments: 'It's allright', 'It doesn't bother me', or 'You have to face it'. Just 6% said they were happy living alone. A further 10% made both negative and neutral comments about it, 4% had mixed feelings, giving both negative and positive responses, and 3% made other comments.

A third, 34%, said they found living alone 'very difficult' to accept, 31% found it 'fairly difficult', and 33% found it 'not difficult', while 2% made other comments. Those who found it difficult made the following types of comment:

'I'm very lonely. I wish I had gone with him. I kiss his photo every night and say "Why did you leave me?". Every time I go into the bedroom I picture him laying there. I don't really like it on my own.'

'There's not much excitement — it's boring all day long. At night I sit down, then I get up and shave and go off hoping to find someone to keep me company. Then I come home again to an empty house.'

'I hate it, I loathe it. I just think it's a terrible way of ending up the last lap of your life.'

'I don't like it. I used to say to him, "Just don't leave me. Never leave me here." At about half past nine when it's getting dark I feel frightened. When he was here I was never frightened. I do miss him so much.'

'It's purgatory living alone. It's sapping my will power and my will to live.'

[1] 'Apart from missing your husband/wife what do you feel about living alone?'

Table 22   Acceptance of living alone and other attitudes and psychological problems

	On balance finds living alone:		
	Very difficult to accept	Fairly difficult to accept	Not difficult
Has problems with:			
Sleeplessness	65%	54%	36%
Nerves or depression	66%	48%	30%
Irritability	23%	8%	7%
Loss of appetite	26%	16%	7%
Finds loneliness:	%	%	%
A big problem	51	28	5
A problem will get over soon	18	29	26
No problem	26	38	68
Other comment	5	5	1
Has come to terms with spouse's death	23%	37%	39%
Does not think will come to terms with spouse's death	64%	16%	16%
Described the way things were going for them as reasonable*	80%	93%	96%
Would like life to continue in much the same way**	62%	76%	85%
Regards home as very convenient	59%	58%	73%
Number of widowed (= 100%)	94	86	89

* 'Taken together would you describe the way things are going for you these days as: "reasonable", "not very well", or "not at all well"?' (adapted from Parkes 1979).

** 'So thinking of how your life is going now, would you wish: "it to continue in much the same way", "to change some parts of it", or "to change many parts of it"?' (also from Parkes 1979).

Forty-three per cent of those living alone felt they had already got used to it, 36% thought they would do so eventually, but 16% did not think they would ever do so. Five per cent made other comments. Naturally those who said they found living alone very difficult to accept were relatively unlikely to say they had already got used to it, but 17% of them felt they had done so, compared with 42% of those who said they found it fairly difficult to accept, and 73% of those who found it not difficult.

Although there were no clear trends with age in the proportion who said they had difficulty in adjusting to living alone, the older widowed, aged seventy and over, were rather more likely to say they had already got used to it: half of them said they had done so compared with a third of the younger widowed. There was no apparent difference between widows and widowers over this.

Experiencing difficulty in adjusting to living alone was associated with a number of other attitudes, emotions, and psychological symptoms. Those who found living alone difficult to accept were more likely to report problems with sleeplessness, nerves or depression, irritability, and loss of appetite. They more often found loneliness a problem and were less likely to think they either had, or ever would, come to terms with their spouse's death. In addition fewer of them felt things were going reasonably well for them or wanted life to continue in much the same way. They were also less likely to regard their home as very convenient. The figures are in *Table 22*.

Apart from these mainly subjective feelings, we did not find any relationship between their acceptance of living alone and such material circumstances as their housing arrangements or equipment, contact with relatives and friends, existence of children, their mobility, or how well they knew their neighbours. However, there was no doubt that those who were finding it difficult to adjust to living alone were more anxious about their financial situation than others. The data are in *Table 23*. In addition to financial anxieties, loneliness, depression, and other emotional problems, there was some indication that those who found living alone difficult to accept may have suffered more from feelings of guilt: almost half, 45%, of those widows and widowers who said they would have liked something done differently before their spouse died said they found living alone 'very difficult' to accept, in comparison with 31% of the other widowed.

The loneliness and insecurity of living alone appeared to be one of the most difficult aspects of widowhood to accept:

> 'I'm not a person who likes to be alone − I just want my husband. I daren't live in the house without a burglar alarm system, I wouldn't sleep without that. During the winter with all that snow nobody came, I was very isolated.'

> 'Well it's the deathly silence. You could die and nobody would know until the paper was left in the door.'

Table 23   Acceptance of living alone and financial anxieties

	On balance finds living alone:		
	Very difficult to accept	*Fairly difficult to accept*	*Not difficult*
Proportion saying money is a problem for them	35%	32%	14%
Proportion who say they are a great deal worse off since their spouse died	20%	22%	6%
Proportion saying there is a problem in relation to expense with their home	45%	24%	19%
Proportion who have or expect to have difficulty keeping warm	22%	10%	8%
Number of widowed (= 100%)	94	86	89

'If I passed out in this house I think it would be days before anyone found me.'

Widowhood and a life alone disrupts routine and the fabric of life:

'I don't like it [living alone]. There's just no-one to talk to when you require it. When you've been used to being a partnership it's a boredom. It's a terrible loss. When I come in from work there was always a fire, my tea ready. I'd change, watch the 5.45 news, then I'd snooze for half an hour. Then we'd have a natter and perhaps go out to see friends. But now I have to do it all, get the meal, clear up, light a fire. You hop into bed and where her bottom would be there's nothing.'

Domestic circumstances

Most of the widowed had lived in their home for some time.[2] Few, 16%, had lived in their present home for less than 5 years, while most, 62%, had lived there for 15 years or more. Two-thirds lived in a complete house, 17% in a bungalow, 16% in a flat or maisonette, and 1% in rooms.

[2] The few who had moved were asked how long they had been living in their previous homes.

Home ownership may often give feelings of independence and security which may be valued at times of loss. Just over a third of the widowed, 39%, owned their home outright and 3% owned it on a mortgage, 40% rented from the council, and the remainder rented privately, 13%, or, in 5% of cases, lived in homes owned by relatives. Those in the middle classes, as may be expected, were more likely to be outright home owners than those in the working classes − 47% in comparison with 29%.

Most, 86%, had four or more rooms in their homes,[3] 95% had their own bathrooms, and 94% had their own indoor lavatories. Because of the difficulties elderly people may experience with steps, we asked about steps and the number of floors in their homes. Two-thirds, 66%, had at least one floor between ground floor level and their bedrooms. About a quarter, 24%, had either a floor or steps between their bedrooms and the lavatory.

Over three-quarters, 79%, felt the size of their homes was 'about right' for their present needs but a fifth said their home was 'too big'. Widowers were more likely than widows to feel their home was 'too big' − 30% compared with 14%, although there were no differences between them in the number of rooms in their home. Two-fifths with six or more rooms thought their home was too big, and this proportion fell to 13% of those with three or four rooms, and none at all of those with fewer rooms. Less than 1% of all the widowed thought their home was too small.

Familiars were more inclined than the widows and widowers to describe the widowed people's home as 'too big' for them now. Thirty per cent of all familiars felt this and this proportion was still 20% when the widows felt it was about the right size.

Wicks (1978), in his national survey of hypothermia, found a sub stantial minority of people aged sixty-five and over either hypo-thermic during the winter or with inner body temperatures so low that they were at risk of developing hypothermia. He found that the vast majority of the elderly lived in rooms with temperatures below recommended levels. The most efficient form of heating was found to be central heating although less than one in four of his sample pos-sessed it. Wicks recommended electric blankets as an effective preventive measure against hypothermia. We asked the widowed about the types of heating they had. Most had more than one sort. Almost half, 45%, had some form of central heating, almost

[3] This included bedrooms, living rooms, and any kitchen or scullery.

three-quarters, 70%, had electric fires, and half had gas fires. Over a third, 37%, had coal or coke fires, 21% used paraffin heaters or oil stoves. Sixty-one per cent had an electric blanket.

Over two-thirds of the widowed, 68%, were satisfied with their heating, although almost a fifth, 19%, complained of the expense, 11% said it was inadequate, and 2% said it was troublesome. No differences were found with type of heating and their satisfaction with it.

Almost a fifth, 15%, said they had, or thought they would have, problems or difficulty keeping warm, and 7% were uncertain about this:

'I was frozen last winter.'

'It was murder — my pension went just on heating.'

Those in the working classes were more likely than those in the middle classes to say they had, or would have, problems, 18% in comparison with 9%. No significant differences with age or sex were found.

We asked about the possession of other domestic appliances. A significant minority lacked equipment which might have made life easier for them. A quarter possessed no washing machine; just over a fifth, 22%, did not have a spin dryer, and 11% did not have a refrigerator. Between 5% and 6% said they would have found these useful. An important piece of equipment, especially when living alone and in declining health, is a telephone. Three-fifths of the widowed had a telephone, and three-fifths of those without one said they would find a telephone useful. The significance of the possession of a telephone for some is illustrated by the following statements:

'If only I had a 'phone, I'd feel I'd got someone.'

'I am happier now there is a telephone in the bedroom. I do get very nervous at night.'

A trend was found with possession of a telephone and social class, varying from 85% of those in Social Classes I and II, to 44% of those in Social Class V.

We asked the widowed whether they would say their home was all right or whether they had any problems with stairs, hot water and other amenities, expense, nearness to shops and to relatives and friends. A third, 31%, mentioned problems with the expense of their home; a fifth, 18%, distance from relatives and friends; 16% distance from shops; 13% had problems with stairs; and 8% had problems with the hot water and other amenities. Most, 64%, described their home as 'very convenient', and 28% described them as 'fairly convenient'. Also when asked openly 'What do you feel about your present home?', 56% made positive comments − for example they said they were happy or satisfied with their home, that it was comfortable, or that they had happy memories. Twelve per cent made neutral comments such as 'It's allright', and 11% made negative comments. Main criticisms were that their home was difficult to manage, or isolated and lonely. A further 11% had mixed feelings about their home, making both negative and positive comments. Similarly, Age Concern's 1974 survey of elderly people found that the majority, 87%, expressed satisfaction with their accommodation. Possibly older people have lower expectations and are more willing to put up with inconvenient aspects of their home. They may also be more attached to them after having spent a large proportion of their lives in them.

Potential movers

A third of the widowed were either thinking of moving or someone had suggested that they might do so, although the majority, three-fifths, thought they would probably stay in their present home for the rest of their lives − leaving 7% who were not contemplating moving but felt uncertain about what might happen eventually:

'It depends how much time I've got left and on being able to manage the garden.'

'Everybody has said to me "Are you going to stay here?". But I haven't thought about moving. This is my home and I will stay. . . . Probably if I get very old and decrepit I will move. You have to be fairly tough to live here, because it isn't all that convenient. You have to be able to drive a car.'

'If ever I become incapable I should go into a home where there was a doctor in charge.'

'If I won the pools I'd be away tomorrow.'

Under what circumstances do elderly widowed people consider moving home? Poor health, inconvenient homes, and homes that were too big for them were factors which appeared to be related to the possibility of moving (see *Table 24*). Working-class widows and widowers were more likely than those classified as middle class to say they thought they would stay in their present home. This did not seem to be because financial restrictions might make moving more difficult for them since no relationship was found here between thinking of moving and money as a problem, or being worse off financially since the death.

Table 24   Those expecting to stay in their present home for the rest of their lives

	Percentage expecting to stay in present home for the rest of their lives	Number of widowed (= 100%)
Health:		
Excellent or good	63%	191
Fair or poor	52%	146
Social class:		
Middle class	46%	91
Working class	61%	254
Regards present home as:		
Too big	45%	67
About right size	62%	268
Present home:		
All right	71%	164
Some problems	46%	176

The proportion who might move was similar for widows and widowers, and there was no clear trend with age. But feelings about their memories were related to their desire to move. We asked those who were still living in the same home as before the death whether the memories associated with their home made them want to move away or stay. Eleven per cent said they made them want to move:

'Everywhere you look you think he's sitting in that chair.'

Most, however, wanted to stay because of the memories:

'I don't want to move. I don't want to leave my hubby — he's here still.'

And whereas only 6% of those who wanted to move because of their memories thought they would spend the rest of their lives in their present home, this proportion was 69% of those who wanted to stay because of their memories.

Shanas, *et al.* (1968) found that elderly people tend to prefer not to live with their relatives. They found that while just 8% of their national sample of elderly people said they preferred to live with children or other relatives, 83% preferred their own home. Just under a third, 30%, of the widowed in the present study who were considering moving said they would be living with someone they knew, while over half, 56%, would be living near but not with someone they knew, leaving 14% who would not have anyone they knew living with or near them. Some mentioned the dilemma of whether or not to live with children and risk disrupting both their lives or the lives of the children:

> 'I wouldn't want to upset my son's home life. Girls and boys should have their own homes and ways of life.'

The elderly may also be reluctant to become dependent on their children feeling this may change the nature of their relationship. On the other hand, stigma or fear seemed to be attached to old people's homes:

> 'I see so many old people and they've gone in there and − perhaps I shouldn't say this − but they're waiting to die. It's the last place you go.'

Among the third who had considered moving, 25% felt it would be more of a disadvantage than an advantage, 57% that it was mainly an advantage, and 15% that the advantages and disadvantages were equally balanced. (A few made other comments.) They were less likely to view the move as an advantage if it meant going to live with relatives − only 42% regarded it as an advantage in those circumstances, compared with 60% in others.

When those who might move were asked what they saw as the main advantages and disadvantages, the main advantages, mentioned by 29%, were having better facilities in the home − such as no stairs, or a smaller, or more modern home:

> 'There'd be less work. This place is falling apart.'

Another 29% said they would be nearer relatives or friends:

> 'I'd be near my daughter. She could do little things I might need help with as I'm getting older.'

Twelve per cent said they would no longer be alone or isolated as they would be living with others:

> 'I wouldn't have the fear of living alone.'

And 11% mentioned better facilities outside the home – such as being nearer the shops. While 16% could see no advantages.

The main disadvantages mentioned by 15% were not knowing anyone or so many people in a different area:

> 'If I went there I'd have to make new friends and at my age I'm not likely to.'

Loss of independence where the move involved sharing with others was stressed by 8%:

> 'Well you like to have your own home and be independent.'

> 'I'd lose my freedom in lots of little ways. They all add up. I prefer to visit [daughter].'

> 'Getting in the way and having rows.'

A variety of other disadvantages were cited, but 50% said there were no disadvantages although there may have been practical problems in arranging the move, since it would involve buying or renting accommodation for most of them. The proportions are shown in *Table 25*.

Table 25   What a move would involve

Type of arrangement:	%
Sharing with relatives	24
Buying	14
Renting from council – exchange	11
Renting from council – other	30
Renting privately	6
Going into old persons' home	4
Other	5
Uncertain	6
Number of potential movers (= 100%)	102

Almost a third, 29%, of the potential movers said someone was trying to persuade them to move — one widow whose sons were trying to persuade her to move into a council house nearer them said:

'My sons say I could walk around —— (town) in the afternoon, but who wants to walk around —— in the afternoon? I would never see a nicer view than I have here.'

Other widows seemed irritated by suggestions of moving:

'My daughter wants me to move in with her but I won't go.'

'Everybody's had me moving into a flat but I don't want a flat.'

'People are always suggesting I ought to move. I'm sick and tired of telling them that I am not going to move.'

One widow even said that the main advantage of the proposed move was to satisfy her daughter:

'It would make my daughter happy. I'd be under her wing.'

We asked the widowed if they had thought at all, or if anyone had suggested, a lodger, or friend or relative, coming to live with them. Nine per cent said this had been considered or suggested but many of these expressed reservations:

'I'd have to be careful, wouldn't I, not to get the wrong sort?'

'I've changed my mind. My sister says they run you in the end — your house ceases to be your own.'

They were also asked whether they were planning or thinking about the possibility of any, or any other changes, in their lives. The majority, 95%, were not. Apart from facing life without their partners, and the emotional upheaval and role re-orientations this may have involved, few life changes occurred after widowhood. Glick, Weiss, and Parkes (1974) found that change was more evident in the lives of younger widows.

Adjusting to new roles

With the death of a spouse people may be faced with taking on new practical tasks which they might never have thought about before. A widow may have lost the person she relied on to do the lifting and other physical jobs around the house, while a widower may have lost the person who looked after him and his home. It is possible that, at a time of stress, as in bereavement, the enormity of such a change in roles becomes magnified and may have some effect on emotional adjustment. Older men and women, in particular, may find it difficult to take on the traditional roles of the opposite sex. These now have to be coped with.

This role change may be especially difficult if the widowed were no fitter than the deceased. Dependence before the death may have been mutual or the widowed person might even have been more dependent on the spouse. Fifteen per cent of the widowed, in reply to a direct question, said the deceased was the fittest of the two of them, and 15% said they were both the same. These widows and widowers may find adaptation particularly difficult, and even the widowed defined as the fittest were sometimes in poor health. Some illustrations:

'We were two poor old things, although I was the fittest at the end.'

'I can't understand why I didn't go first, I was always ill. Yet he suddenly died. One day we were talking and I said "What happens if you go first? I don't know anything about money or anything." When he grinned, I said "Don't you be too clever because one day someone may put a hand on you".'

'He wasn't an ill man. He looked after me all the time. I've had a colostomy — in 1974 — and another abdominal operation in 1975. That caused a hernia and I've got it now.'

'It wasn't him that needed help, he had to do everything for me. I'm the one who needs help.'

'He said "I don't want to leave you". He said to the doctor "I've got to get better to look after my wife and daughter. They're two cripples." The doctor just smiled.'

Widows were less likely than widowers to feel they had been the fittest, 64% against 79%.

Lopata (1971) argues that people who have been recently widowed, especially those who are older, need to be trained to be independent because they are not always able to make decisions and act in the areas in which the husband, or wife, specialized. She calls for the setting-up of special centres with doctors, solicitors, and social workers available to give advice and help to the widowed. To what extent did the widowed in the present study have difficulties taking on new roles? Do these difficulties warrant the establishment of such advice centres or perhaps even a system of screening the bereaved by social workers? How they coped partly depended on the roles adopted within the marriage relationship and whether skills were shared. For example, one widow said:

'He did the lot, that's why I'm lost.'

To what extent were household tasks shared?

Table 26 shows that many of the deceased had performed household tasks.[4] The sex distribution also shows that men more often took on traditional male tasks such as odd jobs and gardening, and women took on the more traditionally female housekeeping role. The only task done with roughly equal frequency by men and women was window-cleaning.

Table 26   Domestic tasks performed by men and women before their illness and death

	Sex of deceased		Both sexes
	Men	Women	
Tasks performed:	%	%	%
Shopping	54	89	66
Preparing/cooking food	38	96	58
Washing up	69	87	75
Making beds	23	93	48
Cleaning house	39	92	58
Washing clothes	16	90	42
Cleaning windows	38	45	41
Gardening	68	28	54
Other odd jobs around house	74	34	60
None of these	6	2	5
Number of deaths (= 100%)	232	126	358

As would be expected from sex-role divisions before the death, sex differences were found with the tasks the widowed started doing. Widowers were more likely to have started doing traditional female tasks such as shopping, preparing and cooking food, washing up, making beds, and washing clothes. Widows were more likely to start

[4] 'Did your husband/wife do any of these household things before he/she became ill/died?'

Table 27   Tasks widows and widowers started doing after the illness or death, tasks they do now, and those they have help with

Tasks performed:	Tasks widowed started doing		Tasks widowed do now		Tasks widowed have help with	
	Widows	Widowers	Widows	Widowers	Widows	Widowers
	%	%	%	%	%	%
Shopping	8	53	82	83	32	36
Preparing/cooking food	4	66	91	84	12	31
Washing up	11	51	95	90	13	19
Making beds	4	71	89	82	9	24
Cleaning house	3	59	87	78	28	48
Washing clothes	1	47	80	54	20	65
Cleaning windows	11	18	64	65	47	47
Gardening	23	9	52	68	45	19
Other odd jobs around house	28	16	51	80	44	20
None of these	47	10	1	4	17	18
Number of widowed (=100%)	197	116	223	125	222	124

doing traditional male tasks such as gardening and odd jobs around the house. The figures are in *Table 27*.

Fewer sex differences were found with tasks the widowed were doing currently, presumably because many of them had to take on the tasks which their partners had done previously. *Table 27* also shows that widowers were more likely than widows to get help with cooking, bed-making, cleaning, and washing clothes while the reverse was true for gardening and odd jobs. Besides window-cleaning, there was no difference in the proportion of widows and widowers who got help with shopping and washing up.

Older widows and widowers got more help with domestic tasks than younger ones: 90% of widows aged seventy-five or more got some help compared with 80% of younger widows, while the comparable figures for widowers were 92% and 75%. And, as would be expected, those sharing their homes were more likely to have help with household tasks than those living alone, 83% in comparison with 50%. To some extent home helps and paid help compensated for some of this difference. Nearly half, 47%, of those living alone had such help compared with 39% of others.

Rainwater (1965), amongst others, found that lower-class couples had a clear differentiation of labour into male and female tasks. In his study, middle classes had less sharply polarized relationships and placed greater value on sharing and on the interchangeability of tasks. He also found a higher degree of joint role organization and equality amongst the upper middle class. On the other hand, it has been found that there is a greater degree of sharing of household tasks following retirement in both social classes, although this is apparently welcomed more by middle-class couples (Kerckhoff 1966). This may explain the fewer social-class differences found in the present study and why we found hardly any social-class differences in tasks done by the deceased (46% of middle-class women compared with 30% of working-class ones were said to have done 'odd jobs around the house'). No differences with social class were found with things the widowed started doing after the death.

Middle-class widows and widowers were more likely to have a home or paid help than working-class ones, 50% in comparison with 39%. Presumably this was mainly private help as few of the widowed said, in reply to a direct question later on, that they had a home help − 16%.

How do the widowed cope with taking on these new roles? We asked them whether they had any problems with the listed domestic tasks. For almost three-quarters of widows, 71%, and widowers, 74%, no problems were reported. Over a quarter, then, reported problems. And a similar proportion said they needed help, or more help, with some of the tasks. Gardening and odd jobs around the house were the tasks most likely to present problems, and they were also most frequently mentioned as the ones they would like some or more help with, by 14% and 9% respectively. Widows were more likely than widowers to need help with odd jobs, 12% in comparison with 5%. There were no other differences with sex. Those in poor health were more likely to have problems with the various domestic tasks. The proportion who said they had no problems with any of them declined from 82% of those who described their health as excellent, to 77% of those in good health, 65% with fair health, and 56% of those in poor health. New tasks may appear overwhelming, especially when no help is available, and when combined with ill-health:

'He'd hoover and wash, clean the inside windows. He was a handy man. I couldn't put a globe on or de-frost the fridge. I've had to learn. I'm frightened I'll fall with the curtains. I'll have to get round to it somehow. I've nobody [to help].'

'I don't feel I'm fit enough. I'm seventy-four. I have never been used to doing these things. I'm afraid I'll fall, I've wobbly knees.'

We asked the 60% who had started doing various household tasks, since the illness or death, how they felt about these. Almost half, 49%, said they liked them, 13% disliked them, and 36% had mixed feelings, 2% making other comments. Widowers were more likely than widows to dislike their additional tasks, 19% in comparison with 8% of widows, but as we showed earlier the jobs they had taken on were very different. The most common new jobs for roughly a quarter of the widows were gardening and odd jobs around the house, while more than half the widowers had started to shop, cook, wash up, make beds, and clean the house. Some widowers regarded the taking-on of new tasks as a challenge, especially now they often had less to occupy themselves with. They became 'something to do'. As one commented:

'If I hadn't got them to do I'd be lost. I'd have nothing to occupy me.'

For widows, in contrast, there was more often a contraction rather than an extension of their household tasks:

'There's not nearly so much to do now he's gone. There's just the gap. That's the trouble.'

'I've not enough to do — I can't find enough to do, even to take me up to 12 o'clock dinner-time.'

But this could happen to widowers too if their wives had been ill for some time. One widower, aged between 65 and 69, whose wife had been ill for twenty years with multiple sclerosis and who retired at 62 to look after her said:

'I've had less to do than for a long time. Over the years I had to do more and more. At first I helped her with the shopping and the housework. I had to do more as she got worse and then she lost the use of her legs. I had a home help when my wife was bad but I telephoned her when she died and said I didn't want any more help because I hadn't enough to keep me going. I clean up after breakfast, go to the shops, get me lunch and that's that — nothing else to do.'

If the deceased was ill for a long time then the spouse may have adjusted to new roles during this period:

'I've got no problems, not like that. It's a long time since my wife could do much. I've got used to doing everything.'

'He was ill for such a long time — he had his first stroke ten years ago — so I've been doing most things since then.'

Widows and widowers were asked about the various role divisions in their marriages, before the illness or death. We asked them what sort of things their spouses did which were most of a problem for them now that they were no longer here to do them. Less than a third, 29%, said no problems had emerged as yet, sometimes this was because they received help. Also, the spouse had sometimes been too ill to do things before the death anyway. The problems most frequently mentioned were financial and business affairs, by 14%; odd jobs around the house, by 12%; household tasks such as making beds, washing, and so on, by 12%; gardening by 9%; cooking by 8%; and 7% mentioned lifting things and other physical jobs, and also decorating and painting. For example:

'All sorts of jobs — lifting and moving things. I can't do it. It's awful when you're left.'

'All the bills, writing, problems to do with finance. I didn't know how he paid his gas bills. It's a great mistake for a wife to leave everything like that to her husband. It worried me when he died. I dreaded to see a buff envelope on the mat.'

'Cooking and washing up and all that. She never stopped, always working.'

'There's a lot of jobs around the house he did which I can't do. He used the hoover, I can't use it very much it's too heavy. He did the lifting, he'd get down and brush the carpet. I can't get up and down. He used to unscrew jars. I haven't any grip. I've had two strokes myself. He put my stockings on when my back was bad. I can't get them on. He used to rub my back with liniment. You can't rub your own back.'

'I don't know how to work the central heating. I've been told and told, but it won't sink in.'

The widowed were asked directly about who had taken care of the business affairs,[5] lifting things and other physical jobs,[6] and the

---

[5] '(So) how did you and your husband/wife divide various jobs between you before he/she became ill/died? Who looked after business affairs such as paying bills, or any insurance — was it you or —— or both equally?'

[6] 'And, who did most of lifting things around and other physical jobs?'

Table 28   Division of tasks during marriage by sex

	Widow	Widower
Business affairs done mainly by:	%	%
Husband	35	31
Wife	48	43
Both equally	16	25
Other answer	1	1
Lifting and physical jobs done mainly by:	%	%
Husband	47	80
Wife	28	3
Both equally	21	16
Other answer	4	1
Planning and decision-making done mainly by:	%	%
Husband	7	10
Wife	14	14
Both equally	78	76
Other answer	1	—
Number of widowed (= 100%)	233	128

planning and decision making.[7] *Table 28* shows the sex-role distributions for these tasks. Perceptions of widows and widowers were
similar for business affairs and planning and decision-making but
differed markedly for lifting and physical jobs. Of course we only
collected this information from the surviving spouse.

Because of traditional sex-role divisions it might be expected that
each of these tasks would have been performed mainly by men, but
this assumption was only supported in the case of physical tasks.
While planning and decision-making tended to be divided equally
between the couple, women were more likely to take care of business
affairs. However, among the middle classes men were more likely to
take care of business affairs, but among the working classes women
were more likely to do this. This difference is shown in *Table 29*.

Possibly in working-class families the man tends to give his earnings
to his wife who controls household expenditure, but in middle-class
families the man controls both income and outgoings. The division

[7] 'What about the planning and decision-making – was that you or ——, or
did you share it equally?'

Table 29   Division of business affairs by social class and sex

	Widows		Widowers	
	Middle-class	Working-class	Middle-class	Working-class
Done mainly by:	%	%	%	%
Husband	59	26	52	23
Wife	24	57	31	48
Both equally	15	16	17	28
Other comment	2	1	–	1
Number of widowed (=100%)	59	171	35	90

of such tasks will affect the extent to which the widowed will have to adjust to a new situation:

'We used to talk everything over. That's what I miss now.'

'She did the lot.'

'He just used to say "You settle the bills, you know where the money is".'

If there is a need for an advice service for the widowed about the business affairs associated with running a home, it is the middle-class widows and the working-class widowers to whom it seems most appropriate to direct it.

Finance

For most people as they get older their income drops. Their dependence on pensions is reinforced as their assets wear out. Further, as health worsens so the need for extra income for heating and other needs may increase. The income and expenditure patterns of the elderly certainly show a marked contrast from those of other households. The DHSS's analyses of the Family Expenditure Survey (1977) show that 46% of elderly families as against 18% of all families live below, at, or no more than 10% above, supplementary benefit level. The death of a spouse may temporarily or permanently worsen the widowed person's financial situation because of the legal formalities, such as the will, which may have to be sorted out, and because of changes in pension rates. When asked whether they had got their financial position sorted out, almost a fifth, 19%, said they had not.

The most common problem tended to be due to delays in receiving benefits — either social security, supplementary benefit, or pensions, or due to delays by solicitors. In reply to a direct question, 11% of the widowed said there had been problems or delays in getting their new pensions or benefits:

> 'I haven't had the pension from the pit yet. When all the bills come in it's a problem.'

For three widows the circumstances of the delay in receiving their benefits were particularly upsetting:

> 'At first they [social security] made out I was dead and sent it to my husband in his name. They did have the decency to apologize. It isn't sorted out yet.'

> 'They addressed it to my husband even after I had written to tell them that he had died and that I was re-applying as a widow. What can you do with people like that?'

> 'They sent giros and even sent my husband a new pension book.'

No differences were found with social class and delays or problems here. When asked about their financial situation, over half, 54%, said they were, or would be, financially worse off after the death; 20% said they were a little worse off, 17% said they were a moderate amount worse off, 16% said they were a great deal worse off, and 1% made other comments. The widowed generally felt they were worse off because they now had only one pension instead of two, and the outgoings were similar:

> 'My pension has come down to about £30 a week instead of £40 when my husband was alive. The rent of the flat costs £15 so there's not much left.'

> 'There is less money coming in and you still have to pay the same big expenses, rates, heating, coal, and all that.'

Almost a fifth, 17%, of those who said they were worse off said they went short of things they needed, usually clothes, food, and heating. We also asked whether money was a problem for them — 30% said it was:

> 'It's a problem when you get the phone bill or electric. When it's

cold the money all goes on coal, and when you want new clothes it's a problem.'

Those classified as working class were more likely to say that money was a problem, 33% in comparison with 20% of the middle class.

To what extent was money a problem to the widowed because their financial position had deteriorated since their spouse's death? The relationship between the two is shown in *Table 30*. Deterioration is clearly a substantial part of the problem but not the whole of it. The middle-class widowed were as likely as working-class ones to say they were worse off financially, and the proportion describing themselves as a great deal worse off also did not vary with social class. So this sort of relative deprivation, unlike finding money a problem, was not related to class.

Table 30   Money a problem and changes in financial position

	Widow or widower is or will be:			
	A great deal worse off	A moderate amount worse off	A little worse off	No worse off
Money a problem:	%	%	%	%
Yes	67	35	31	10
No	33	65	69	89
Other comment	–	–	–	1
Number of widowed (= 100%)	55	60	68	131

Sources of income and other benefits are shown in *Table 31* together with social-class differences. Old age pensions were the most common source of income and there was no class difference in the proportion receiving this. The middle class were more likely to have other retirement pensions while more of those in the working class were on supplementary benefit, received rent rebates, and had help from social services with heating. The middle class were as likely as the working class to take advantage of the cheap rail pass but more of the working class had bus passes. They were also more likely to receive help from their relatives.

When asked whether there was anything they felt to be a particular problem in their present lives, 15% said 'money'. More, 41%, said

Table 31 Sources of finance and other benefits by social class

	Middle class	Working class	All widowed
Source:	%	%	%
Old age pension	80	77	78
Other retirement pension	53	37	41
Widow's pension	12	15	14
Private insurance	9	6	7
Supplementary benefit	11	36	29
Rent or rate rebate	30	48	43
Help from social services with			
Telephone	1	2	2
Television	–	3	2
Heating	5	13	11
Cheap rail-pass	14	13	13
Cheap bus-pass	54	70	65
Help from relatives	3	14	11
Other financial help	8	3	4
None of these	3	3	3
Number of widowed (= 100%)	91	253	347

there was something they would like to do or have if they had a bit more money to spend. The thing most often mentioned, by 17% of all the widowed, was holidays; 6% said household goods and equipment.

Diet

About a tenth, 11%, of the widowed, in reply to a direct question, said they did not think they had a proper diet. Just over half of these said this was because they could not be bothered. One widow who said she kept her husband alive with the nursing care she gave him for eighteen months, now expressed feelings of wishing to die herself:

'Some days I feel like throwing the sponge in.'

About her diet she said:

'I don't eat very well, I just don't want to be bothered.'

Cooking for friends and relatives often gave the widowed more incentive to eat properly themselves:

'Sometimes you want to cook something or eat something and I can't be bothered. But my friend comes on Monday, Wednesday, and Friday and she clears the rooms for me and says "We'll have so and so and you cook it for us".'

About a twelfth, 8%, had either meals on wheels, meals at a luncheon club, or, where these services were unavailable, received luncheon vouchers from social security. The majority of these, 84%, had between two and five meals a week with these systems. When asked whether they would like any, or any more of these meals, 3% said yes. Most tended to comment that they did not fancy them:

'I've seen some. Have you seen what they offer the old people? No thank you, not for me.'

'I don't think I would be able to cope with their kind of cooking.'

For 12% of the widowed, relatives, friends, or neighbours brought in meals. For 3% they were brought daily, for another 3% more than weekly but less than daily, for 4% weekly, and the remainder received them less often.

The majority of widows and widowers, 78%, had been invited out to meals by relatives, friends, or neighbours since the death. Two-fifths were invited out more now, for a third the frequency was about the same, while one in twenty were invited out less now. There were no differences between these widowed people in terms of sex, age, or social class. Of those who were not invited out to meals now, almost a fifth, 19%, said they, and their spouses, were asked out before the illness or death. Many of these widows and widowers stopped going out during the illness, and the social isolation continued after the death. For some, however, widowhood meant the beginning of greater isolation. As one widow commented:

'We had friends [but] as soon as a woman loses her husband people think you won't want to go out. Nobody wants a widow.'

Loneliness was indeed a common problem and is discussed later in Chapter 7.

Summing-up

The most frequent practical problems facing these elderly people in the months following their widowhood were adapting to living alone, coping with new household tasks, and adjusting to a lower income.

While many widowers were facing the need to shop and cook for the first time in their lives, widows had to cope with a more negative change: shopping and cooking just for one.

A third were considering the possibility of moving, but only one in twenty had actually moved in the five months following the death. For the most part they valued their independence and were reluctant to relinquish this by going to live with relatives or friends. Although one in three had a home which they found inconvenient in some way, most of the widowed had lived in their homes for ten or more years, and they were attached to their homes and the memories associated with them. After the trauma and upheaval of widowhood few were planning other major changes in their lives.

Money problems, reported by nearly a third, accentuated other difficulties: 79% of those who had such problems and were now living alone said they were finding this difficult to accept, compared with 61% in that situation but without money problems. In later chapters we show how financial problems relate to other difficulties.

5 Health and the role of the general practitioner

The health problems of the elderly widowed are likely to have been exacerbated by the practical and emotional strains of caring for their husband or wife in the weeks, months, and often years before their spouse's death. Then there will have been the trauma of the death itself, after which the majority were faced with the problem of learning to live alone, while substantial proportions had to cope with financial stringency and the problems of new tasks and responsibilities.

In this chapter we are concerned with the elderly widowed's health problems and with the part that general practitioners did and could play in helping them to cope with and adjust to their new situations. We start by looking at their contacts before the funeral.

Contacts between the widowed and their general practitioners before the funeral

When the general practitioners were asked what they thought they should do when an elderly patient (of pensionable age) was widowed, the most common view, held by 41%, was that they should visit the elderly widowed at home. Thirty-six per cent said it would depend entirely on the circumstances, while 15% thought they should just respond to direct requests for help, leaving 8% who felt they should contact the widowed, possibly by letter or telephone, to see if he or she needed a doctor's help. Those who said it depended on the circumstances were asked to say in what circumstances they thought a general practitioner should initiate a visit. Several said they should do so if there were no close relatives or friends to give support. Other circumstances they mentioned were if the widow or widower was emotionally disturbed, if he or she was physically unfit, if there was a close relationship between the doctor and the widow or widower, or if the death was unexpected.

Most doctors, 64%, thought that if a general practitioner was to contact an elderly patient who had been widowed, the doctor should do this as soon as possible; 10% thought it should be done a few days after the death, but before the funeral; while 20% thought it should be soon after the funeral, and 4% some time later. (Two per cent made other comments.) General practitioners learnt about two-thirds of the deaths of their married patients within twenty-four hours and of four-fifths within three days. (For further details see Cartwright 1982.)

However the majority of the widowed, two-thirds, had not seen a general practitioner after their spouse died but before the funeral. *Table 32* shows that general practitioners who thought they should visit were more likely than others to do so, but even then half the widowed had not seen their general practitioner before the funeral.

Table 32   Relationship between the doctors' views and the experience of the widowed

	Doctor feels that when an elderly patient is widowed the general practitioner should:		All widowed
	Visit them at home	Depends on circumstances, or other answer	
Widow or widower saw general practitioner before funeral:	%	%	%
At home	45	18	24
At surgery or elsewhere only	4	10	10
Did not see general practitioner	51	72	66
Number of widowed (= 100%)	53	79	349

There was no difference in the proportion of widows and widowers who saw a general practitioner before the funeral, but among those who had seen a doctor more widows than widowers had been visited at home, 78% compared with 55%, while a higher proportion of widowers went to the surgery, 38% against 14% (a few had been seen elsewhere). Most of those who had seen a doctor saw their own general practitioner; one in eight of those who did not have any contact with their own doctor during that time said they would have liked to have seen their doctor then. One widow said:

> 'I 'phoned the surgery and spoke to the receptionist and she said if I sent someone up she would give them some Valium for me. My daughter got them and they did help but I would have liked to have seen the doctor and talk about things.'

Three-fifths of the widowed who had seen a doctor after the death but before the funeral were given a prescription. Widows were more likely to have been given one than widowers, 68% compared with 49%.

There was some evidence that the general practitioner was more likely to give a prescription at this point in time if he or she had had relatively little contact with the person who died. The proportion of widowed given a prescription at that time declined from 77% of those whose spouse had no home visits or just one visit from a general practitioner in the year before their death, to 61% of those whose spouse had from two to nine home visits, and to 48% of those whose spouse was visited ten or more times.[1] Of the widowed who described the general practitioner's care of their spouse as 'very good' 52% were given a prescription, compared with 76% of those who described it as 'fairly good' or as 'not very good'. If we accept the assessment of the widowed person it would seem that the less caring doctors are more likely to prescribe pills for bereavement.

Those who were given a prescription were less likely to describe their relationship with their doctor as friendly[2] than those who were not given one, 47% compared with 67%. And those who were given a prescription appeared less likely to regard their doctor as easy to talk to − 86% compared with 95% of those who were not given one − but this last difference might have occurred by chance.

[1] These percentages, and the others in this paragraph, relate only to the widows and widowers who had the same doctor as their spouse who died.

[2] 'Do you consider your doctor to be something of a personal friend or is your relationship pretty much a businesslike one?'

96   Life After A Death

The health needs and problems of the widowed

The widowed were asked if they regarded their health for their age as excellent, good, fair, or poor. Their responses are shown in *Table 33* alongside the replies of two random samples of people aged sixty-five or more. The widowed were less likely to rate their health for their age as excellent, but on the other hand, compared with one of the studies, relatively few rated it as poor. As they have survived their spouse they may feel that their health cannot compare too badly with that of others of the same age; at the same time the strains and stresses of the bereavement, on top of coping with the terminal illness of their husband or wife, is likely to leave them feeling less robust than others without that experience.

Table 33   Widows' and widowers' estimates of their health 'for their age' compared with estimates of a random sample of people aged 65 or more

	The widowed	Random sample aged 65 or more	
		Cartwright and Anderson (1981)	Dunnell and Cartwright (1972)
Health for age rated as:	%	%	%
Excellent	14	26	22
Good	42	42	38
Fair	35	25	27
Poor	8	7	13
Other comment	1	–	–
Number of people (=100%)	352	165	274

Were any circumstances related to their spouse's death associated with widoweds' assessments of their health? Whether they reported the death as expected or not did not appear to be associated with their view of their health at the time of interview, nor did their estimate of the length of time their husband or wife had been ill before the death. But the proportion who said their husband or wife had been mentally confused increased from 20% of those who described their own health as excellent to 44% of those who reckoned it was poor. And those who

Table 34 Symptoms reported by the widowed and by a random sample of people aged 65 or more

	Proportion of people aged 65+ reporting symptom in a two-week period	Proportion of the widowed reporting problems with symptoms	Proportion of symptoms that developed since, or became worse after, spouse's death*	
	%	%		
Breathlessness	21	37	36%	(131)
Indigestion or stomach trouble	23	30	24%	(106)
Headaches	22	28	35%	(97)
Backache	21	39	17%	(137)
Rheumatism, etc.**	41	59	27%	(208)
Sleeplessness	22	50	65%	(176)
Trouble with teeth or gums	4	9	45%	(33)
Corns, bunions, or trouble with feet	34	33	18%	(114)
Nerves or depression }	15	47	72%	(163)
Irritability }		14	48%	(50)
Forgetfulness or confusion	***	43	53%	(150)
Loss of appetite	6	17	83%	(59)
Any difficulty seeing	***	23	41%	(80)
Any difficulty hearing	***	31	30%	(110)
Other problem		8	0%	(27)
No problem		5		
Number of people (= 100%)	280	350	*All symptoms* 41%	(1641)

* Figures in brackets indicate the numbers on which the percentages are based.
** Rheumatism or aches or pains in the joints, muscles, arms, or legs.
*** Not asked about.

rated their health as only fair or as poor were more likely than the others to say they wished something could have been done differently before their spouse died. The proportion who wished this was 30% for this group compared with 18% for those who rated their health as excellent or good. In contrast those with better health were *more* likely to be critical of the way the general practitioner had looked after their spouse before the death;[3] the proportion who described the general practitioner's care as 'not very good' declined from 20% of those with excellent health to 4% of those with poor health. Possibly those with less good health felt more dependent on the doctor and were less willing to criticize him or her.

Comparing the symptoms the widowed reported with those reported in an earlier study by a random sample of people aged 65 or more (Dunnell and Cartwright 1972), we found that for the symptoms asked about in both studies — breathlessness, indigestion, headaches, backache, rheumatism, sleeplessness, trouble with teeth or gums, trouble with feet, nerves or depression, and loss of appetite — the widowed reported eight out of ten of them more frequently. The two exceptions were headaches and trouble with feet (see *Table 34*). But the widowed were asked whether they had any problems with the symptoms while the other study asked about symptoms in a two-week period.

The most common symptoms reported by the widowed were rheumatism, sleeplessness, nerves or depression, and forgetfulness or confusion. Over two-fifths were suffering from each of these. Two-fifths of the symptoms they reported were said to have developed since, or become worse after, their spouse's death. The highest proportion of symptoms falling in this category were loss of appetite, nerves or depression, sleeplessness, forgetfulness or confusion, and irritability. Few backaches or foot troubles were classified in this way. It is possible that these symptoms may have been exacerbated by nursing their spouse during their last illness and some may have improved since the death.

Two-fifths of the widowed had some problems of mobility and looking after themselves. The nature of these problems is shown in *Table 35*. One in six either could not or had difficulty going out, a fifth were unable to or had problems getting in and out of a bath, and stairs presented problems to a quarter. Widows were considerably more likely to have mobility problems than widowers and, as might be expected, the proportion with such problems rose sharply with age, from 20% of those under 60 to 70% of those aged 80 or more. In contrast there were no appreciable differences between widows and widowers in their health ratings, nor were there any clear trends

---

[3] 'How do you feel about the care and treatment —— had from his/her general practitioner before his/her death?'. 'So would you say it was good, fairly good, or not very good?'.

Table 35 Problems of mobility and personal care

	Widows	*Widowers*	*Both sexes*
Widow or widower cannot, on own:	%	%	%
Use public transport	14	3	11
Go out	8	–	5
Go up and down stairs	6	2	5
Get in and out of bath	6	2	5
Dress and undress	–	–	–
Cut toe nails	16	12	14
Widow or widower can only with difficulty:			
Use public transport	12	8	11
Go out	11	10	11
Go up and down stairs	26	12	21
Get in and out of bath	19	8	15
Dress and undress	8	4	7
Cut toe nails	19	15	17
Widow or widower has some other problem of this sort	5	8	6
No problem	52	71	59
Number of widowed (= 100%)	228	124	352

related to age. Differing expectations and standards presumably accounted for this lack of difference.

As can be seen from *Table 36* more widows than widowers reported problems with headaches, backache, rheumatism, sleeplessness, their feet, nerves or depression, and loss of appetite, but then in general more women than men report these problems (Dunnell and Cartwright 1972). There was no indication that more of the widows' than of the widowers' problems were attributed to their widowhood.

Forgetfulness or confusion and difficulties with seeing and hearing increased with age. Problems with sleeplessness on the other hand were reported more often by those under 70 than by those aged 70 or more: 57% against 45%. For the other symptoms there were no clear trends or significant differences. This may be partly due to changing expectations and different tolerance levels. There were no social-class variations in the widows' and widowers' reports of their health problems.

Table 36   Variations in symptoms reported with sex and age

	Sex		Age					
	Widows	Widowers	Under 60	60–64	65–69	70–74	75–79	80+
	%	%	%	%	%	%	%	%
Breathlessness	38	36	36	35	35	39	37	43
Indigestion or stomach trouble	29	32	28	22	26	30	35	39
Headaches	32	20	20	22	39	28	32	10
Backache	45	29	48	38	41	29	45	45
Rheumatism, etc.*	64	52	68	62	51	56	68	63
Sleeplessness	57	38	52	54	60	48	46	39
Trouble with teeth or gums	10	8	8	19	10	6	11	6
Trouble with feet**	36	26	28	19	36	32	42	29
Nerves or depression	53	35	56	49	50	46	42	41
Irritability	14	15	12	19	20	11	9	16
Forgetfulness or confusion	43	42	28	32	45	41	51	49
Loss of appetite	21	10	16	8	25	18	14	12
Any difficult seeing	24	20	16	8	25	20	28	33
Any difficulty hearing	27	39	8	14	29	25	45	57
Other problems	8	7	4	8	10	10	3	8
No problem	4	6	8	5	4	5	3	4
Average number of problems	5.0	4.1	4.3	4.1	5.0	4.4	5.1	4.9
Number of widowed (=100%)	226	124	25	37	80	93	65	49

* Rheumatism or aches or pains in the joints, muscles, arms, or legs.
** Corns, bunions, or trouble with feet.

Health and some social circumstances

The widowed who lived alone were no more healthy than those who lived with others. So it did not seem as if their own ill-health had been a reason for sharing a home with relatives or friends. If anything, those who lived by themselves rated their health for their age as rather *less* good than those who lived with other people: 45% of those living alone rated their health as fair or poor, 37% of the others — a difference which might have occurred by chance. Neither was there any significant difference between those living alone and the others in terms of their mobility, problems with personal care, or in the symptoms they reported.

But there was some suggestion that those who felt themselves to be in good health may have been somewhat less likely than those with fair or poor health to be contemplating moving in the future. The proportion who thought they would probably stay in their present home for the rest of their lives declined from 67% of those with excellent health to 52% of those who rated their health as fair or poor. Only 4% of those who might move were thinking of going into an old person's home. One reason why those in less good health might be more likely to be thinking of moving was that they were less likely to regard their home as very convenient for them, and more of them reported problems with it. The data are in *Table 37*.

Since health was closely related to mobility (the proportion reporting no problems on that score fell from 84% of those who rated their

Table 37   Health and housing

	Widow or widower regarded health for age as:				All widowed
	Excellent	*Good*	*Fair*	*Poor*	
Described present home as:	%	%	%	%	%
Very convenient	74	67	62	44	64
Fairly convenient	20	29	29	37	28
Rather inconvenient	6	3	9	15	7
Other comment	–	1	–	4	1
Reported problems with home with:	%	%	%	%	%
Stairs	6	6	16	48	13
Hot water and other amenities	6	3	10	26	8
Expense	24	22	40	44	31
Nearness to shops	8	14	19	26	16
Nearness to relatives and friends	16	11	22	37	18
Other problems	2	1	2	–	1
No problems	60	60	36	7	48
Number of widowed (=100%)	50	149	124	27	352

health as excellent, to 15% of those who described it as poor), it is not surprising that those with less good health would report more problems with stairs and accessibility. Those with mobility problems were less likely than other widows or widowers to have any stairs or steps between the front door and their bedroom (62% of them had some stairs or steps, compared with 77% of those with no mobility problems), but there was no difference between the two groups in the proportion who had stairs or steps between their bedroom and the lavatory: this proportion was 24%.

At first sight it may seem less understandable why those with only fair or poor health perceive more problems in relation to the expense of their housing than those with good or excellent health. The most plausible explanation is that the sick need more money. Whether or not they were worse off financially since their spouse died was *not* related to their assessment of their health; neither was the extent to which they were worse off. But the proportion who said they went short of something they needed was 3% among those with good or excellent health, 15% among those with fair or poor health; the proportion who said money was a problem for them rose from 21% of those with excellent health to 44% of those with poor health; and the proportion who had, or thought they would have, difficulty keeping warm rose from 4% of those with excellent health, to 24% of those who described their health as fair, and to 44% among those who regarded it as poor.

Contact with general practitioners

As we have seen only a minority of the widowed had any contact with a general practitioner before their spouse's funeral but, by the time we saw them, some five or six months after their spouse had died, the majority had had at least one consultation with a general practitioner. The details are in *Table 38*. It is possible to make a crude estimate of the average number of consultations from the figures in *Table 38*. For all consultations this comes to 2.55 or the equivalent of 5.65 for a full year. This compares with an average of 4.02 for a random sample of people aged sixty-five or more taken from the electoral register (Cartwright and Anderson 1981).

The extent to which the widowed's contact with general practitioners varied with their health is shown in *Table 39*. There was a stronger association with home visits than with total consultations.

Table 38 Contacts with general practitioner during the five or six months after their spouse's death

	All consultations	*Home visits*	*Consultation with own general practitioner*
	%	%	%
None	24	67	34
One	25	17	24
Two–four	37	13	31
Five–nine	9	2	7
Ten or more	5	1	4
Number of widowed (= 100%)	350	340	348

There were no significant variations in total consultations or home visits with sex, and total consultations did not vary significantly with age, within this limited age range. But the proportion with a home visit was much higher for those aged 75 or more: 61% compared with 30% of those under 75. If some older people cannot get to the surgery on their own and so only see the doctor when he or she visits them, this may explain why the total consultation rate did not increase with age. If anything, those living alone were *less* likely to have seen a doctor than those living with others after their bereavement, 74% compared with 82%, but this difference might have occurred by chance. There

Table 39 Variation in contact with general practitioner and health

	Widowed's rating of own health for their age:			
	Excellent	*Good*	*Fair*	*Poor*
Average number of contacts since spouse's death:				
Total consultations	1.9	2.2	3.0	3.5
Home visits	0.5	0.8	0.9	2.4
Proportion who saw a doctor before funeral	20%	30%	40%	52%
Number of widowed (= 100%)	50	149	124	27

were no significant variations with social class, nor by whether the widow or widower had any children. In fact consultations were clearly related to health and to mobility but *not* to social problems such as living alone, or having housing or financial difficulties. Those who said they suffered from nerves or depression were more likely to have seen a general practitioner than those who did not report these symptoms, 84% against 69%, but this means that 16% of those who were depressed had not been in touch with a doctor since their bereavement.

But even if the majority of those who reported nerves or depression had seen a doctor at some stage since their bereavement, they had not necessarily talked to the doctor about this. When asked whether they had consulted a doctor about particular symptoms, half said they had done so about their nerves or depression, only just over half, 55%, about their hearing difficulties, and a similar proportion about sleeplessness. A third said they had told a doctor about their lack of appetite, fewer still, 15%, about their confusion or forgetfulness — but of course some may have forgotten or been confused about this.

When asked why they had not consulted a doctor about particular symptoms, only a few gave reasons for not consulting the doctor at all:

'I didn't want to send for him and I can't go down [to the surgery].'

More frequent reasons were that they felt they did not want to bother the doctor about the symptom:

'I don't like complaining. I've had many things.' (Not consulted doctor about difficulty seeing or difficulty hearing.)

Or they thought it would get better on its own:

'I've never bothered to. I think it will get better.' (Not consulted doctor about sleeplessness.)

'It will get right. I don't want to be addicted to pills.' (Not consulted about sleeplessness.)

Several mentioned a reluctance to take pills:

'I don't want to take sleeping tablets.' (Not consulted about sleeplessness.)

'He'd only give me sleeping tablets and I don't want such things as that.' (Not consulted about sleeplessness.)

'Because I don't want pills.' (Not consulted about nerves or depression.)

Other comments were:

'Something you've got to expect in later years.' (Not consulted about forgetfulness or confusion, or about difficulty seeing.)

'I keep away as long as I can.' (Not consulted about difficulty hearing.)

'I've got to do it myself.' (Not consulted about nerves or depression.)

In another study (Cartwright, Hockey, and Anderson 1973) it was found that an important reason for not consulting the doctor about particular symptoms was a realistic assessment of the inability to help with certain symptoms. The same probably holds here for forgetfulness or confusion, irritability, and loss of appetite. But probably the most disturbing finding is that nearly half the widowed had not consulted a doctor about difficulty with hearing. This was apparently accepted as an inevitable part of ageing without first checking that a doctor could do nothing to alleviate the problem. The widowed were more likely to have consulted a doctor about nerves or depression and sleeplessness than about irritability and confusion − almost certainly because of expectations that the doctor could prescribe something that might alleviate the first group of symptoms. The question of medicine taking is considered next.

Medicine taking

Over three-quarters of the widowed said they had taken or used some prescribed medicine, tablets, or ointments since the death of their spouse, and nearly two-thirds, 63%, had taken some prescribed medication during the two weeks before they were interviewed. In spite of their relatively high consultation rate this last proportion was similar to that in a general sample of people aged sixty-five or more who were taking prescribed medicine in 1977 (Anderson 1980a). But of course many medicines are taken on repeat prescription (Anderson 1980b), and 31% of the widowed who had not consulted a general practitioner since their spouse's death had taken some prescribed medicine in the two weeks before they were interviewed.

However *psychotropic drug* taking was more common among the elderly widowed than among a general sample of similar ages

Table 40   Types of prescribed drugs taken by the elderly widowed compared with those taken by a random sample of people aged 65 or more

	Proportion of the widowed taking drugs		Proportion of random sample aged 65+ taking drugs in two weeks before interview
	Since death of spouse	In two weeks before interview	
Type of drug:	%	%	%
Psychotropic			
Minor tranquilliser			
sedative or hypnotic	32	24	
Major tranquilliser			
sedative or hypnotic	3	3	
Anti-depressant or			
stimulant	5	3	
Other	1 (37)	1 (28)	(20)
Other nervous system	14	12	9
Gastro-intestinal	13	10	4
Cardiovascular/diuretic	26	25	28
Respiratory/allergic	6	5	9
Rheumatic	11	9	10
Anti-microbial	9	3	4
Endocrinological	5	4	8
Nutrition/blood	5	3	4
Skin/eye/mucous			
membrane	6	5	6
Other	1	1	1
Name of preparation not			
known	6	2	1
None	22	37	43
Number of people (= 100%)	351	350	163

Percentages add to more than 100 as some people were taking more than one type of drug.

(Cartwright and Anderson 1981, additional unpublished data). Over a third, 37%, of the elderly widowed had taken some type of psycho-tropic drug since the death of their husband or wife and 28% had taken them in the two weeks before the interview. Most of the psycho-tropic drugs that they were taking, 83%, were classified as minor tranquillizers, sedatives, or hypnotics. Three per cent of the elderly widowed were taking major tranquillizers and 4% were on anti-depressants. In addition to psychotropic drugs a relatively high proportion of the widowed were taking gastro-intestinal drugs. The proportions taking different types of drugs are shown in *Table 40*. For details of the way in which they have been classified see Appendix VI. It is clear that quite a number of widowed people were given psychotropic drugs in the period immediately after their bereavement. This may be seen as an indication that as Illich (1974) claims some doctors seek to remove the human capacity to experience pain. But some of the widowed may well have been exhausted and in need of a good night's sleep.

The length of time since they first got a prescription for the various types of drug is shown in *Table 41*, together with the proportion who were still taking the drugs in the two weeks before they were interviewed. Compared with most other types of drugs apart from those operating on infections and for respiratory conditions, the psychotropics were relatively likely to have been prescribed since the spouse's death. But three-quarters of the psychotropics were being taken in the two weeks before interview. A further analysis showed that of those psychotropic drugs first prescribed since the spouse's death, 59% were

Table 41   Prescribed medicines taken since spouse's death by when first obtained a prescription, and whether taken in the two weeks before interview

	Psychotropics	Other nervous system	Gastro-intestinal	Cardiovascular and diuretics	Respiratory	Rheumatism	Infections	Skin/eye/mucous	Other	Not known	All drugs
First obtained prescription:	%	%	%	%	%	%	%	%	%	%	%
Within month before interview	8	16	12	3	14	10	16	11	12	5	9
Since death but more than 1 month ago	41	24	30	12	36	24	45	29	24	59	30
Before death but less than 1 year ago	15	18	22	19	4	6	10	11	17	8	15
1 year but less than 5 years ago	18	24	18	38	21	31	3	28	21	15	24
5 years or more ago	18	18	18	28	25	29	26	21	26	13	22
Proportion taken in the two weeks before interview	74%	82%	80%	92%	80%	81%	39%	75%	74%	45%	76%
Number of drugs (=100%)	156	50	50	154	28	49	31	28	42	61	649

Table 42   Conditions for which prescribed medicines taken

	Medicines taken:			
	Since death of spouse		In two weeks before interview	
	%		%	
Infective and parasitic	2		1	
Endocrine, nutritional, and metabolic	4		5	
Diseases of blood	2		1	
Diseases and symptoms of circulatory system	17		21	
Bronchitis	2		2	
Other respiratory diseases and symptoms	8		7	
Digestive/gastro-intestinal diseases and symptoms	7		7	
Genito-urinary	4		5	
Skin diseases	3		3	
Musculo-skeletal diseases and symptoms	14		14	
Mental disorders, nervousness, debility	28		24	
Nerves or depression		10		7
Sleeplessness		14		14
Nervous system and sense organs – diseases and symptoms	2		3	
Other symptoms, ill-defined conditions	7		7	
Number of medicines (= 100%)	623		467	

still being taken in the two weeks before interview. Not surprisingly a higher proportion, 87%, of those prescribed earlier were still being taken.

The conditions for which medicines were taken are shown in *Table 42*. Roughly a quarter were taken for mental disorders including nerves or depression and sleeplessness. Details of the classification of conditions are given in Appendix VII. An analysis of the proportion of all drugs taken at any time since their spouse's death that were taken in the two weeks before interview shows that 56% of those who had taken some prescribed medicine for nerves or depression were still taking it, compared with 74% who were still using their drugs for sleeplessness.

One of the dangers of taking psychotropic drugs is that it may become a habit. An intention to help people through a difficult period of adjustment may develop into continuing support. This is particularly true for bereavement which has no clear end point and the period of distress may last for some considerable time. In some ways it may seem surprising that minor tranquillizers were prescribed so much more often than anti-depressants, given the high proportion reporting problems with nerves or depression and the increased likelihood of bereaved people developing a depression that leads to mental hospital admission (Parkes 1964).

Who takes the medicines?

Not surprisingly the average number of medicines taken in a two-week period was highly correlated with the widowed's assessment of their health, rising from 0.6 for those who described their health as excellent to 3.1 for those who rated it as poor. But although widows reported more health problems than widowers, there was no difference between the sexes in the average number of medicines they were taking. This is consistent with Anderson's (1980a) findings on medicine taking in relation to men and women aged sixty-five or more. These findings suggest that widows were less likely to be taking some medication for a particular problem than widowers. There was however no clear evidence that they were less − or more − likely to consult a doctor about particular problems. The widowed over seventy were taking more medicines than the younger widowed; the average numbers during the last two weeks were 1.6 and 1.1 respectively. There were no social-class differences.

Some of the widowed were not taking the medicines the doctors had prescribed for them: twenty of them, 6%, said, in answer to a direct question, that since their spouse's death they had been prescribed some medicine that they had not taken. One of these had only just got two medicines and had not had time to start taking them. Five had in fact taken a little of the medicine but stopped because of side effects:

'They were for my nerves − to help me not to cry. They didn't suit me. They made me annoyed and bad-tempered. I only took two.'

Three had not needed them yet, including one who had been prescribed glyceryl trinitrate for angina but who had not had an attack since she got the tablets, another who had been given Valium:

'in case I get too much depressed. I haven't needed them, I'm keeping them in case.'

while the third had been given sleeping tablets and said

'I don't like to [take them]. I know they are there if I really need them.'

Six others had been given sleeping tablets but 'did not believe in them'. Some of their comments were:

'I prefer whisky. I have a quirk against them.'

'I don't believe in drugs. When you hear of all the side effects − I'd rather not sleep.'

'I've tried to do without them. I thought I might become addicted to them.'

Two of the three who had been given drugs for their nerves but had not taken them referred to the dangers of addiction:

'I'm afraid to get hooked on something you can't get off.'

'I don't want to start a habit with them.'

The third who had been given tranquillizers told us:

'My daughter said as soon as she saw them "Throw these away". So I did − down the toilet.'

The remaining two who had not taken their prescribed medicines also did not like the idea of taking drugs. One had been given pills for a pain in the neck:

'I just felt the stiff neck would go away without the pills. I am anti-pill. I thought he would have sent me for heat treatment.'

The other who had been given tablets for rheumatism said simply:

'I don't like taking tablets. I'm allright really.'

All except one of the twenty had got their prescription made up. The other, whose doctor had given her some sleeping pills directly, 'chucked them in the dustbin'.

Who is taking which medicines?

Earlier we showed that widows were more likely than widowers to have been given a prescription or drugs before the funeral. In addition widows were more likely than widowers to be taking psychotropic drugs: 45% compared with 25% had taken such drugs since their spouse died. It was the minor tranquillizers, sedatives, and hypnotics which accounted for this difference: 41% of the widows, 20% of the widowers had taken these. Similar proportions of the two sexes, 5%, had taken anti-depressants, and 2% of widows compared with 4% of widowers major tranquillizers − a difference which might well occur by chance. Rather more men than women had taken preparations acting on the respiratory system or affecting allergic reactions: 1% against 4%.

It was the younger widowed, under 65, who were more likely to be taking minor tranquillizers: 48% of them had done so, 32% of those aged 65 or more. This relates to a finding reported later, in Chapter 7, that the younger widowed more often reported problems with loneliness. The proportion taking any type of psychotropic drug was 48% among those who said that loneliness was a problem for them,[4] 28% among those who felt it was not. The proportions taking minor tranquillizers, sedatives, and hypnotics were 44% of the lonely, 23% of the others. The taking of preparations acting on the gastro-intestinal system increased with age from 5% of those under 65 to 21% of those aged 75 or more, and cardiovascular and diuretic drug taking was more common among those aged 65 or more, 30%, than among the younger widowed, 18%. The types of drugs the widowed were taking did not vary with their social class, but the working class were less likely to know the name of the drugs: 2% of the middle class compared with 7% of the working class had taken prescribed drugs they were unable to identify. (Names of drugs are written on the bottles but some were no longer being taken and the bottles had been thrown away.)

The widows' and widowers' views of their general practitioners

The widowed who had seen their own doctor since their spouse died were asked whether they had found their doctor very sympathetic, fairly sympathetic, or rather unsympathetic. Two-thirds said very

[4] 'What about loneliness − do you find this a problem for you or not?'

Table 43   Views on sympathy and other attributes of their general practitioner

	Found general practitioner:			Own general practitioner not consulted since spouse's death	All widowed
	Very sympathetic	Fairly sympathetic	Not very sympathetic		
Considers relationship with doctor:	%	%	%	%	%
Friendly	58	33	10	36	43
Businesslike	39	63	90	62	54
Uncertain – a bit of both	3	4	–	2	3
Thinks doctor:	%	%	%	%	%
Easy person to talk to	98	91	33	81	87
Not easy	2	7	62	17	12
Other comment	–	2	5	2	1
Thinks doctor has time to discuss things:	%	%	%	%	%
Yes	94	66	24	69	77
No	5	28	71	26	19
Other comment	1	6	5	5	4
Number of widowed (=100%)	147	46	21	115	345

sympathetic, a fifth fairly sympathetic, a tenth rather unsympathetic, and the rest made other comments. The ways in which their perceptions about this were related to their assessments of other attributes of their doctor are shown in *Table 43*. Sympathy is strongly related to a friendly relationship, being easy to talk to, and having time to discuss things. Those who had not consulted their doctor since their bereavement had rather similar views about him or her as those who had found their doctor to be 'fairly sympathetic'. Those who described their relationship with their doctor as friendly were more likely to prefer it the way it was than those who said their relationship was more businesslike. Only 1% of those who said it was friendly would prefer it to be more businesslike but 19% of those who said it was businesslike would prefer it to be more friendly.

Apart from presumably feeling happier and more relaxed with a doctor they found to be sympathetic, did that aspect of their relationship affect the number and nature of their contacts with their doctor?

Whether or not they found their doctor very sympathetic did not' vary with the number of consultations they had had, nor with the number of prescribed medicines they were currently taking, but those who reported problems with nerves or depression were more likely to have discussed this with their doctor if they regarded him or her as sympathetic: the proportions were 82% of those who found their doctor very sympathetic, 72% of those who found him or her fairly sympathetic, and 62% of those who thought their doctor 'rather unsympathetic'. And earlier we showed that this was related to whether or not they had discussed their spouse's illness or possible death with their doctor. Of course it may be that having raised such issues with the doctor they found the doctor to be sympathetic, but then the implication is that something in the doctor's manner or attitude can encourage or enable elderly people to discuss such problems.

In spite of the fact that the widowed who regarded their doctor as sympathetic were more likely to have consulted him or her about their nerves or depression, those who found their doctor 'rather unsympathetic' were more likely to have taken minor tranquillizers than those who described him or her as very or fairly sympathetic. In contrast, it was those who found their doctor 'very sympathetic' who were most likely to be taking cardiovascular or diuretic drugs. The figures are in *Table 44*. There were no differences with other types of drugs, or with other attitudes.

Some idea of the sort of help and support people appreciated from their general practitioner comes from the two who mentioned their

Table 44   Views on sympathy and drug taking

	Widowed found general practitioner:		
	Very sympathetic	Fairly sympathetic	Rather unsympathetic
Since spouse's death had taken prescribed:			
Minor tranquillizer	39%	43%	62%
Any psychotropic drug	44%	49%	67%
Cardiovascular or diuretic drug	38%	26%	29%
Number of widowed (= 100%)	148	47	21

doctor as the only person whom they had found helpful to talk to[5] after their husband or wife died. Both of these were widowers. One lived on his own and said:

> 'The doctor has done more than anyone else to help me. He's a fantastic man — a genuine Christian.'

But although he said he found the doctor extremely easy to talk to and had seen the doctor two to four times since his wife died, he had not consulted him about his nerves or depression, forgetfulness or confusion, and lack of appetite from which he had suffered since his wife died because:

> 'I found it difficult to talk about them. In fact at the time I wasn't able to mention it.'

The other lived with a handicapped daughter and had been very ill with influenza and bronchitis after his wife's death. He said about his doctor:

> 'He's as friendly as can be. . . . He stays there in the room as long as you want him to.'

Even so he had not yet consulted his doctor about his hearing which had 'gone very bad over the last six months'. But he intended to see his doctor about it.

At the other end of the scale were the nine widowed (4% of those who had consulted a general practitioner since their spouse's death) who said they did not feel they had had enough, or the right sort of help from their doctor since their spouse had died. One widower in his late seventies had nursed his wife who had Parkinson's disease for eight years before she went into hospital less than a month before she died:

> 'I fed her, cut her nails, did her hair, and wiped her when she was messy. I couldn't get her in and out of the bath. I washed her down in a bowl. She couldn't do anything for herself. I had to put her on the lavatory. I did it all myself. She was my wife. It's the natural thing to do.'

He described his own health as 'terrible' and said he couldn't walk any distance because of his legs which were swollen and ached terribly.

[5] 'When someone close to you dies who do you feel it is best to talk to about how you feel?'. 'Who, if anyone, did you find most helpful?'.

Since his wife's death he had seen a general practitioner once, after he had asked him to call at home:

> 'He told me off for sending for him. He walked in and said "I thought you were dying by the message I got". I felt real bad. That's no way for a doctor to talk to a patient. He talks as if he's the top dog and you're nothing.'

He suffered from sleeplessness, loss of appetite, and difficulty hearing, as well as the trouble with his legs which had got worse recently. But he had not consulted his doctor about any of these:

> 'How many doctors would listen? – It wouldn't do any good, he'd say I was wasting his time.'

And about the deafness, 'He would say it's my age'. His sister who now lived with him said:

> 'I wish he would see the doctor but he can't get to the surgery himself and the doctor told him off when I asked him to call here.'

He was currently taking three medicines all initially prescribed two or more years previously at a hospital. His sister collects the prescription from the surgery.

Another widower, also in his seventies, who had nursed his wife through a stroke was clearly angry with his doctor:

> 'I hope I never see him again.'

After his wife died

> 'I broke down in health. I had a rash, I knew it was nerves but he told me it was my wrist watch. Did you ever hear such rubbish! I was boiling I don't know how he gets away with it. He just won't stay. He spends two minutes then off he goes. The whole village knows, I don't know why I shouldn't say.'

Part of his anger seemed to stem from the doctor's treatment of his wife:

> 'I was fighting for my missus. It was 24-hour constant attendance for me. They didn't come for eight weeks. He'd come in just for her blood pressure and never listen to her ticker. He could have come more often. I was coping allright so they didn't come.'

A lack of support during his wife's last illness had resulted in an effective breakdown of this man's relationship with his doctor.

The main complaint of one widow was:

'He doesn't really listen to me. My back has been strained in the past, lifting my husband. He says I've been in a draught. He doesn't seem to want to know. He says it's all in the mind. He is always writing things when you're talking. I wonder if he is really listening to me. I'm sure he isn't.'

When asked what her doctor had done for her since her husband died, she said:

'Not very much except give me a lecture and tell me I shouldn't take the tablets for my nerves. He says he doesn't believe in them.'

This widow had been on diazepam for five or more years. It was first prescribed by a hospital doctor.

Another widow declared:

'I haven't a good word for doctors.'

She described her own doctor as:

'A lazy fellow – you can't get him out of his chair. When you go there you just get your five minutes and then it's out and time for the next person.'

This was the widow who had had a colostomy five years before and also had a hernia. She was currently taking four lots of prescribed medicines, but said 'the home help always collects the prescriptions, I just 'phone through'.

A widower had had one visit from his doctor since his wife died; this was before the funeral:

'It was just a courtesy visit. He wasn't here more than a minute. He said I ought to get out of the house, that it was too big for me.'

At this visit the doctor had prescribed 'some vitamins' – Fesovit – which the widower was still taking having obtained a second prescription without seeing the doctor.

These criticisms came from a small minority, but there is some evidence that the widowed may have been reluctant to express criticism of their doctor, when their familiars, on the other hand, felt it reasonable to do so.

Views of the familiars

Twelve per cent of the familiars (three times as many proportionately than of the widowed) felt that the widowed had not had enough or the right sort of help from their doctors since the death of their spouse. Five of the twenty familiars involved said the widow or widower had not seen a doctor at all since the death of their spouse, but the familiars thought a doctor could have helped them. One neighbour and friend who called in every day to see the widower aged 80–84 commented:

> 'His doctor never came to see him after his wife died. I think he should have come to see if he was allright. You don't know what the shock does to them.'

For two daughters, their negative comments about the doctor's care of their fathers (the widowers) seemed, in part at any rate, a spill-over from their feelings about the way the doctor had cared for their mothers who died. One said the doctor had done nothing for her father but:

> 'He [her father] went to see him soon after mum died to tell him – to complain about his not coming out the night before she died. She had this terrible cough. I wanted to get the doctor but she wouldn't have him. Eventually we said take no notice of mum – get the doctor. Dad rang and said the receptionist said doctors don't come out any more. She said come round and I'll give you a prescription. She [the receptionist] made it out. He picked it up and when I phoned dad he said don't worry she seems better. She took anti-biotics that night. During the night he heard a noise and tried to wake her but he couldn't. So he called the emergency doctor and they took her into hospital but it was too late. That doctor had known her for years and years. He knew she must be bad for us to call him. They should know who is genuine and who not. She never bothered anybody. [When dad went afterwards] the doctor said the receptionist hadn't told him that dad had phoned. He said he was very sorry and asked dad if he was sleeping allright. Dad said "What do you think after fifty years?". But he wouldn't have any sleeping pills. He didn't want them. I am not saying he [doctor] could have saved her if he'd come but at least he could have tried. Doctors do come out so that receptionist lied.' (Story essentially the same as widower's.)

The other said:

'I don't think the doctors treat the old people at all well. I think the doctor should have visited him afterwards and I don't think he was very sympathetic the night my mother died.'

Earlier she had said that her mother

'collapsed suddenly in January. The doctor was called, he diagnosed a virus and said she would be all right in 24 hours. In fact she died two hours later.'

Much of the criticism related to the doctors' unwillingness or failure to visit. Another daughter in daily contact with her mother described her mother's care in this way:

'He's only seen her once − when she fell over − her legs went. He gives her tablets for depression and she has had tablets for a heart condition over a long period. He *could* have called to see whether she needed any help. You need someone then if only to say that things are going right. We muddled through without any help but I really think there should be some after-care.'

Yet another daughter said:

'He wouldn't come to see my mum after my dad died, and when she went to see him he was abrupt with her so she walked out of the surgery. The doctor brought her back and he was allright then.'

A niece said:

'I think a visit from a doctor would do more good than anything. She's had a lot of trouble − I've felt really sorry for her and it's been a job to get the doctor to come down. They say "Can she not get here?".' (Widow aged seventy-seven, can only get out with difficulty.)

And another daughter:

'The doctor called to see him the day after my mum died. He said he would call again but he hasn't. I think it would reassure him if his GP saw him occasionally.'

One of the other criticisms also came from a daughter:

'The doctor says they're overworked but I think it's lack of interest. Three months after mother's death the doctor said to him "How is your wife getting on?" – That's group practice for you – still he was the doctor he always sees. Can you imagine?'

This last widower had described his doctor as 'fairly sympathetic'.

In general, the widowed themselves were less critical of the doctor than were the people in closest contact with them. Elsewhere we have shown that most widows and widowers get a great deal of help and support from relatives and friends. The comments in this last section suggest that the widowed may be reluctant to criticize their doctors, and have low expectations about the help and support they might receive from their general practitioners. Their familiars are more prepared to criticize, and some feel that they are left to care for their elderly widowed parents, relatives, and friends without appropriate support or the knowledge that they can turn to the doctor for medical help when it is needed.

Care from other professionals

The majority of general practitioners now have health visitors and nurses attached to their practices, and in 1977 nearly a quarter said they had a social worker (Cartwright and Anderson 1981). So general practitioners might delegate some of the care of their elderly widowed patients to these other professionals. We asked the widows and widowers whether they had been visited at home since their spouse's death by a district nurse (14% said they had), or health visitor (10%), another sort of nurse (2%), or a social worker (13%). Altogether 31% had been seen by one or more of these professionals. The proportion receiving such visits was clearly related to the widowed person's age, health, mobility, and amount of contact with their general practitioner. This can be seen from *Table 45*. But the widowed who lived alone were no more or less likely to have had such a visit, and contact with these services was unrelated to such problems as isolation, loneliness, or financial difficulties. So these services too did not seem to be supporting those with social problems.

Conclusion

The health problems of the elderly widowed are in many ways similar to those of other elderly people, but they are accentuated by loneliness and difficulties in adjustment to their altered status. Probably

Table 45   Visits from a health visitor, nurse, or social worker by various characteristics of the widowed

	Proportion who reported such a visit	Number of widowed (= 100%)
Age:		
Under 60	8%	25
60–64	19%	37
65–69	25%	79
70–74	35%	93
75–79	34%	65
80+	47%	49
Own health for age rated as:		
Excellent	22%	50
Good	25%	149
Fair	40%	121
Poor	37%	27
Any problems with mobility:		
Yes	44%	142
No	22%	207
Consultations with general practitioner since spouse's death:		
None	24%	85
One	22%	88
Two–four	33%	128
Five or more	55%	47
Sex:		
Male	35%	124
Female	28%	225
Lived alone:		
Yes	30%	271
No	33%	78

because of this they are more likely to suffer from nerves and depression, sleeplessness, and lack of appetite, and certainly these are the symptoms they most often attribute to their bereavement. Their health problems are also exacerbated by inappropriate housing and financial difficulties.

Their general practitioners however do not seem to be responding to their social needs and in general these doctors play little part in identifying or easing their difficulties. This conclusion is based on the following findings:

1 Three-fifths of the general practitioners did not feel it was always appropriate for them to visit an elderly patient when he or she had just been widowed.

2 Two-thirds of the elderly widowed had not seen a general practitioner after their spouse died but before the funeral; a higher proportion, three-quarters, had not had a home visit during this time.

3 A tendency to prescribe pills rather than give supportive care to the bereaved was suggested by the findings that the widowed who had found their general practitioner 'rather unsympathetic' were *more* likely to be taking prescribed psychotropic drugs than those who described their doctor as sympathetic. Earlier we showed that general practitioners prescribed pills for the widowed person *more* often immediately after a death if they had *not* visited the spouse at all frequently before the death, and they prescribed pills *less* often if the widow or widower felt the general practitioner's care of their spouse had been 'very good'.

4 A third of the elderly widowed had no contact with their own general practitioner during the five or six months after they were widowed, and two-thirds had no visit from any general practitioner during this time.

5 Whether or not a widow or widower had any contact with a general practitioner was unrelated to the existence of such problems as living alone, housing, or financial difficulties.

At the same time few of the elderly widowed were critical of their general practitioners. Two-thirds of those who had seen their general practitioner since their spouse's death said the doctor had been 'very sympathetic'; three-quarters thought their doctor had time to discuss things; and nearly nine out of ten found him or her easy to talk to. Rather more of the familiars were critical of the care given by the general practitioners to these patients. The evidence from the few widows and widowers who were directly critical of their doctors illustrates the inadequacy of the support given by some doctors and the powerlessness of patients in that situation.

6 General practitioners' knowledge, perception, attitudes, and characteristics

In the last chapter we looked at the ways in which the care received by the widowed from their general practitioners related to their circumstances and problems. In this one we look at certain characteristics of the general practitioners and their attitudes and practices, to see whether these are associated with the type of care given to the elderly widowed. But first we consider their knowledge.

Knowledge

How much do general practitioners know about their elderly widowed patients and their circumstances? To try to answer this we compared the doctor's knowledge about the widows' and widowers' household circumstances and children, with statements made by the widowed. But, in interpreting the results, we should remember that the doctors who completed the questionnaire about individual patients seemed to have a closer relationship and more contact with their elderly widowed patients than doctors who did not complete this questionnaire. In general, then, doctors may be somewhat less well informed about their patients' circumstances than our data suggest.

Eight per cent of the general practitioners indicated that they were uncertain whether their elderly widowed patients lived alone, 83% were right in that their assessment coincided with the information given to us by the widowed, 9% appeared to be mistaken. Of the widowed who lived alone, the doctors believed that 6% lived with others and were uncertain about the position for 7%.

When asked whether the widows and widowers had sons and daughters, 30% of the general practitioners indicated that they did not know the position, 53% gave the correct answer, 17% the wrong one. If the widow or widower had a daughter the general practitioner was aware of this in 79% of instances, but if he or she had a son the general practitioner only realized this in 63%.

There are a number of reasons why general practitioners might not be aware of their patients' home circumstances and family relationships, but it might be expected that the doctors would have reliable records about consultations. However a fifth of the doctors who completed the individual patients' records made no estimate of the total number of consultations the widowed person had had between the death of their spouse and the date of interview. (The two dates were recorded on the questionnaire before it was sent to the doctors and they were asked to indicate whether the widowed had had none, one, two to four, five to nine, or ten or more consultations.) A higher proportion, 28%, made no estimate of the number of visits. It is possible that some of the general practitioners had filled in the questionnaire without referring to the patients' notes.

We had predicted that agreement between the estimates from the general practitioners and the widowed would be less good over home visits than over total consultations and that the widowed would report more home visits than the general practitioners, whereas with total consultations the discrepancies would be more evenly balanced. We made this prediction on the basis of previous experience (Cartwright 1963), and on the assumption that doctors would be less likely to record home visits as they sometimes would not have the records available then. In fact the correlation coefficient of the estimates from the two sources was slightly lower over total consultations, at +0.51, than over visits, +0.69. But over total consultations there was little difference between the estimated means from the two sources – 3.26 against 3.24 – while with the visits, the average based on the doctors' estimates was, if anything, higher than that based on the patients': 1.72 compared with 1.25. Doctors may feel they are making more home visits than they actually do.

Again looking only at the widowed for whom information was available from both sources: 81% of those widowed said they had taken some prescribed drugs since their spouse's death, whereas only 57% of them were said by the doctors to have taken any during this time – and the doctors were specifically asked to include any given

Table 46 Comparison of prescribed drug taking reported by widowed and by general practitioner

	Patient reported taking prescribed drugs since death of spouse		
	Yes	*No*	*Total*
General practitioner recorded widowed as:			
Taking prescribed drug	54%	3%	57%
Not taking prescribed drug	27%	16%	43%
Total	81%	19%	129 = 100%

	Excluding those for whom general practitioner uncertain about consultations		
	Patient reported taking prescribed drugs since death of spouse		
	Yes	*No*	*Total*
General practitioner recorded widowed as:			
Taking prescribed drug	60%	3%	63%
Not taking prescribed drug	22%	15%	37%
Total	82%	18%	101 = 100%

on a repeat prescription.[1] These data suggest that 27% of widowed patients were taking prescribed drugs when the doctor did not realize it, while 3% said they had not taken any drugs although the doctor reported prescribing them. Lack of awareness of drugs prescribed by a hospital cannot account for much of this discrepancy, since 87% of the prescribed drugs taken by the widowed were first prescribed by a general practitioner and of those first prescribed by a hospital 97% were currently taken on repeat prescrption. Another possibility is that

[1] In making this comparison we have excluded the thirteen widowed people who reported taking some prescribed medicine but were said by the general practitioners not to have had any consultations with a general practitioner since their spouse's death, as we did not ask the doctors about medication for this group.

Table 47 Prescribed medication reported by general practitioners and by the elderly widowed themselves

	Proportion of widowed taking drugs since bereavement		
	Reported by widowed	Reported by general practitioners	Reported by both
Types of drugs:			
Psychotropic	%	%	%
Minor tranquillizer, sedative or hypnotic	32 ⎫	21 ⎫	16
Major tranquillizer	3 ⎬ 38	3 ⎬ 29	2
Anti-depressant or stimulant	7 ⎪	5 ⎪	3
Other	1 ⎭	– ⎭	–
Other nervous system	11	2	1
Gastro-intestinal	13	2	2
Cardiovascular/diuretic	26	19	13
Respiratory/allergic	5	5	2
Rheumatic	13	4	3
Anti-microbial	5	5	1
Endocrinological	5	4	3
Nutrition/blood	9	2	1
Skin/eye/mucous membrane	7	2	–
Other	2	–	–
Name of preparation not known or not recorded	9	9	–
None	19	43	16
Number of widowed (= 100%)	129		

doctors did not consult their notes. So we made another comparison, this time excluding those patients for whom the doctors had made no estimate of their number of consultations. The two sets of figures are given in *Table 46*. There are rather fewer discrepancies in the second set, but the implication is that at least a fifth of the widowed were taking prescribed drugs when the doctor thought they were not taking any. Arcand and Williamson (1981) reported a similar discrepancy. In their evaluation of home visiting of patients by physicians in geriatric medicine, they state that a valuable discovery was that 23% of patients were taking drugs not mentioned by the general practitioner.

The types of drugs reported by the widowed and by the general practitioners are compared in *Table 47*. The two distributions were

similar for anti-depressants, major tranquillizers, and endocrino-
logical drugs, but cross-analysis revealed substantial discrepancies.
This is indicated by comparisons with the figures in the last column of
the table. If the information from the widowed people themselves is
accepted, it would seem that doctors were only aware of about half of
the patients who were on minor tranquillizers. The discrepancy was
greatest for rheumatic preparations and there was some suggestion
that patients may have been under-reporting, or not taking, anti-
microbial drugs, but this might be because these drugs were no longer
being taken and the container had been thrown away so they could
not be identified.

In an attempt to identify possible reasons for the discrepancies, we
looked up the questionnaires of the widowed patients who had
reported taking minor tranquillizers which were not recorded by their
doctors. The twenty patients reported taking twenty-three minor
tranquillizers. Prescriptions for six of these twenty-three had first
been obtained two or more years earlier, but for all these six the
patient had had at least ten prescriptions, so it did not seem as if they
were just odd drugs that had been prescribed long ago and then taken
at a time of crisis. Those for which only one prescription had been
given had all been obtained since the death of their spouse. For three-
quarters the prescription had first been obtained from their own
general practitioner, three from another general practitioner (all
these patients had doctors who worked in a partnership). The two who
first got the prescription from a hospital had both had repeat prescriptions; one of them, who had first got a prescription two to five
years previously, said he had had at least forty prescriptions. There
was a possibility that a relatively high proportion of the repeat prescriptions in this group had been obtained without seeing a doctor −
67% compared with 45% of all repeat drugs, but the numbers were
small and the difference might have occurred by chance.

For two-thirds of these patients the doctors recorded that no drugs
had been given since their bereavement, for the others only non-
psychotropic drugs were recorded.

Perceptions

So far we have been looking at factual questions. But in assessing the
sort of care and support elderly widowed patients may get from their
general practitioners, it is also relevant to ask how far their perceptions

of problems and issues are similar or in what ways or directions they differ.

Assessments of the widows' and widowers' health for their age are shown in *Table 48*. There were no people at the two complete extremes with one assessing their health as 'excellent' and the other as 'poor'. However three of the widowed regarded their health as fair when the general practitioner described it as excellent. One of these, a widow, described herself as having had heart attacks and a coronary while her doctor said she had 'mild hypertension'. Another whose doctor reported no health problems or symptoms said she had problems with breathlessness, indigestion or stomach trouble, headaches, backache, rheumatism, sleeplessness, nerves or depression, and irritability.

Table 48 Assessment by general practitioner and widowed of the health of the widowed for their age

	Assessment by widowed:		All widowed
	Excellent or good	Fair or poor	
General practitioners' assessment:	%	%	%
Excellent	20	4	13
Good	51	35	43
Fair	29	52	40
Poor	–	9	4
Number of widowed (= 100%)	69	68	137

At the opposite end, there were six who described their own health as excellent while the general practitioner rated it as only 'fair'. In fact the symptoms identified by these widowed people and their general practitioners often tallied and the difference in the ratings seems to reflect the low expectations of the widowed. For instance one, said by the general practitioner to be frail with early senile changes and to have problems with breathlessness, rheumatism, sleeplessness, and forgetfulness or confusion, herself reported backache, rheumatism, sleeplessness, and forgetfulness, but still regarded her health for her age as excellent. So did another who reported problems with indigestion, backache, sleeplessness, nerves or depression, forgetfulness, and difficulty hearing, while her general practitioner reckoned she had problems with backache, nerves or depression, and hearing.

Overall, however, the general practitioner rated the widowed people's health as better than they did themselves in 31% of instances, as worse in 22%, and they made the same rating on the four-point scale for 47%. To help interpret the differing perceptions of the doctors and the widowed we can put them alongside the perceptions of the familiars. On health, the widowed and the familiars had similar distributions — it was the general practitioners who tended to rate the health of the widowed as rather better.

The general practitioners were asked whether the widows and widowers who were their patients had any problems with ten of the same symptoms that the widowed had been asked about. Replies are compared in *Table 49*. Comparison of the first two columns shows merely whether general practitioners were any more or less likely to complete a questionnaire about the widowed reporting the various symptoms. There were no significant differences.

However there are substantial differences between the second and third columns showing that the widowed were much more likely to report symptoms, than were their general practitioners to regard

Table 49 Symptoms reported by widowed and general practitioners

	Reported by all widowed	Reported by widowed for whom GP completed questionnaire	Reported by GP as present	Proportion of symptoms of which GP was aware	Proportion with symptom according to GP but not to widowed
Breathlessness	37%	42%	16%	28% (54)	5%
Backache	39%	42%	20%	29% (56)	8%
Rheumatism*	59%	63%	35%	45% (86)	5%
Sleeplessness	50%	51%	21%	34% (67)	4%
Nerves or depression	47%	46%	27%	38% (61)	10%
Irritability	14%	16%	5%	13% (23)	2%
Forgetfulness or confusion	43%	46%	8%	10% (60)	4%
Loss of appetite	17%	13%	8%	11% (18)	6%
Any difficulty seeing	23%	21%	6%	18% (28)	2%
Any difficulty hearing	31%	32%	8%	19% (42)	2%
Number on which percentages based (= 100%)	350	142	133		133

* Rheumatism or aches or pains in the joints, muscles, arms, or legs.

them as problems. This is not too surprising. The symptoms of which the general practitioners were most likely to be aware were rheumatism or aches or pains in the joints, muscles, arms, or legs, nerves or depression, and sleeplessness. Backache and breathlessness came next. They were least aware of irritability, loss of appetite, and forgetfulness or confusion. In contrast, the familiars were aware of similar proportions of symptoms as the widowed, except that they were *more* likely to say that the widowed had problems with irritability (26% of them reported that compared with 14% of the widowed themselves).

One obvious reason for the general practitioners' lack of awareness about some symptoms was that the widowed had not specifically consulted their doctors about them. This was discussed in the previous chapter where it was shown that nearly half the widowed had not consulted a doctor about difficulty with hearing. Here we see that the general practitioners were only aware of this problem for a fifth of those who reported it to us. Possibly problems are less likely to be recorded in the notes if nothing is prescribed for them. We did not ask the doctors whether they kept problem-orientated records; it would have been useful to see if those who did differed less from the widowed in their awareness of these problems.

Finally the last column of *Table 49* shows the proportion of the widowed whom the general practitioner perceived as having the various symptoms although the widowed themselves did not report them. It is probably reassuring that so few were seen as having problems with irritability and forgetfulness or confusion. Nerves or depression was the most common diagnosis to be made by the doctor but not the patient. As with sleeplessness, these diagnoses may be related to the prescription of drugs, and if the drugs worked patients may no longer have perceived a problem.

In general, however, it seems as if general practitioners are unaware of a number of health problems faced by their elderly widowed patients and that probably in consequence their overall assessment of the widowed people's health is somewhat better than that which the widowed made themselves.

Housing

In contrast to their perceptions of health, the doctors seemed to rate the housing arrangements of the widowed as rather less suitable than the widowed felt them to be. Only 51% of the housing was rated as 'very suitable' by the general practitioners, whereas 63% of the same widowed people regarded their housing as 'very convenient'. Many of the widowed appeared to be strongly attached to their home and it is likely that the two assessments were made on rather different bases. Different values and expectations about housing are not unexpected as most patients come from a lower social class than their doctors. The association between the two assessments (by the doctors and the widowed) was small and did not reach a level of statistical significance. The familiars perceived the housing and related problems in similar ways as the widowed − as far as the distributions were concerned − the one exception was that rather more of the familiars thought the home was too big for the widowed: 30% compared with 20% of the widowed thought this. The general practitioners were not asked about this.

Loneliness

If there was little or no agreement between the widowed and their doctors in their assessment of their housing, it is hardly surprising that there was no association in their assessments of the widowed people's feelings of loneliness. Half the widowed assessed by the general practitioners said loneliness was a problem for them. When general practitioners were asked whether they thought loneliness was a problem for the widowed their responses fell into three roughly equal parts: for a third they were uncertain, for just under a third they thought it was a problem, and for just over a third that it was not. But although the two distributions were not dissimilar the agreement on individuals was no better than might arise by chance. In contrast there was a strong association − although by no means complete agreement − between the widowed and their familiars on reports of loneliness for the individuals (see Bowling, in draft).

Diet

When asked whether they thought the widow or widower had an adequate diet, the general practitioners were uncertain about a fifth and expressed anxiety about only two (less than 2%). Both of these widowed people realized that their diet was inadequate. In addition, 8% of those whose doctor thought their diet was adequate did not regard it as so themselves, neither did 7% of those whom the doctor was uncertain about.

Mobility and personal care

Over this, general practitioners were most aware of the problems the widowed reported with going out — although if one accepts the widows' and widowers' assessments it might be more appropriate to say the doctors were least unaware of these problems, because they were aware of just over half, were uncertain about a fifth, and did not think there was a problem for the other three-tenths. The doctors were most likely to deny that a problem existed over going up and down stairs, while positive awareness of a problem was least for difficulties getting in and out of the bath, cutting toe nails; the doctors being most uncertain about these. The figures are in *Table 50*.

Table 50   General practitioners' awareness of problems reported by widowed

	Widow or widower reported problem with:				
	Using public transport	*Going out*	*Going up/down stairs*	*Getting in or out of bath*	*Cutting toe nails*
General practitioner:	%	%	%	%	%
Aware of problem	39	52	33	19	18
Uncertain	30	19	14	38	38
Thought no problem with that	31	29	53	43	44
Number of widowed (= 100%)	33	27	43	32	45

The lack of awareness did not seem to arise just because of different standards. For a number of patients the doctor perceived a problem which the widowed did not report. Thus when the doctor said the widow or widower needed help or had problems using public transport, 38% of the widowed said they could do so on their own without difficulty. The corresponding proportion for going out was 26%, for going up and down stairs 18%, and for cutting toe nails 20%. The base numbers are small.

Attitudes

In other studies (Cartwright 1967; Cartwright and Anderson 1981) we have found that general practitioners vary in their estimates of the proportion of their consultations which they feel are for trivial, unnecessary, or inappropriate reasons, and that their estimates relate to circumstances of their work and to their relationships with their patients. In this study too doctors who felt that a small proportion of their consultations were trivial, inappropriate, or unnecessary had a wider view of their work: more of them felt they should contact elderly widowed people to see if they are in need of help, and that they should give elderly widowed people some supervision. Few of them thought that relatives of elderly patients commonly shelved their responsibilities, more of them than of their colleagues who classified a higher proportion of their consultations as trivial would like to give more time to recently widowed patients, and more felt it was appropriate for people to seek help from their general practitioners with problems in their family lives. In addition they were less likely to use a deputizing service. The figures are in *Table 51*. Another difference between the doctors who regarded half or more of their consultations as trivial and the others was that more of the former thought that elderly widowed people should always be offered a sedative: 18% of them felt this, 5% of other doctors. Overall 9% thought this, 45% thought they should 'generally be offered a sedative', 46% that they should 'only exceptionally' be offered one.

However the doctors' estimates of the proportion of trivial consultations were not related to the widowed people's views of their general practitioners.

Most doctors, 75%, thought elderly patients were *less* likely than younger ones to consult for 'trivial' reasons, 6% thought they were more likely, the rest that there was no difference.

The doctor's age

Younger doctors were less likely to be working on their own than older doctors: the proportion who were single-handed declined from 28% of those born before 1927, to 20% of those born between 1927 and 1936, and to 8% of those born in 1937 or later. In spite of this the widowed with younger doctors were more likely to have seen their own doctor since the death of their husband or wife: this proportion

Table 51   Relationship between general practitioners' estimates of the proportion of 'trivial' consultations and their attitudes to other aspects of their work

	Estimated proportion of 'trivial' consultations				All general practitioners
	Less than 10%	10% < 25%	25% < 50%	50% or more	
When elderly person of pensionable age is widowed feels should:	%	%	%	%	%
Visit them at home or contact to see if need doctor's help	74	57	41	39	49
Just respond to direct requests for help	4	6	13	29	15
Depends entirely on circumstances	22	37	46	33	36
Feels elderly bereaved patients should be given some supervision by their general practitioner for a while:	%	%	%	%	%
Generally	59	40	38	31	39
Rarely	–	4	8	17	8
Depends on circumstances	41	56	54	52	53
Thinks relatives of elderly people often shirk their responsibilities and leave it to services to look after old people	19%	29%	46%	52%	38%
Would like to give more time to recently widowed patients	67%	56%	58%	43%	55%
Feels it is appropriate for people to seek help from their general practitioners for problems in their family lives	93%	90%	75%	63%	79%
Uses deputizing service for nights or weekends:	%	%	%	%	%
Regularly	14	23	42	52	35
Occasionally	18	15	19	17	17
Never	68	62	39	31	48
Number of doctors (=100%)	28	48	48	52	176

increased from 58% of those whose doctor was born before 1917 to 75% of those whose doctor was born in 1937 or later. And the average number of consultations rose from 1.72 to 2.88 over the same range. In addition the widowed with the oldest group of doctors − born before 1917 − were least likely to have had a home visit: 20% compared with 35% of the others, although this last difference did not reach a level of statistical significance. But that difference and the others are consistent with findings from another study in relation to the doctor's age, partnership, and consultation rate (Cartwright and Anderson 1981). There were a number of other suggestive differences, in the same direction but not reaching a significant level, indicating that those with an older doctor may have a less close relationship. Among those with a doctor born before 1917 who had seen him or her since their bereavement, 52% said they had found their doctor 'very sympathetic' compared with 67% of the widowed with younger doctors; 20% of the former group did not find their doctor easy to talk to compared with 11% of the others, and the proportions who had talked to a general practitioner about their spouse's illness and what was likely to happen were 47% and 61% respectively. But there were no such differences over whether they found their doctor had time to discuss things or regarded their relationship as friendly or businesslike.

The general practitioners' assessments of the health of the widowed for their age was clearly related to their own age: 68% of the older doctors, born before 1927, regarded the health of the widowed as excellent or good, compared with 46% of younger doctors. As in another study of general practice (Cartwright and Anderson 1981), there was no association between the age of the doctor and the age of the patients. Younger doctors may equate old age with ill health or have different expectations of old age.

Turning to their attitudes to their role, younger doctors appeared to favour more open communication with an elderly person with a terminal illness who asked directly 'Is this going to kill me doctor?'. The proportion who reckoned they would probably give a truthful answer to this rose from 50% of those born before 1927 to 70% of those born in 1937 or later. When asked who they thought was usually the best person to tell a married person that they were unlikely to recover more of the younger doctors mentioned the spouse (26% of those born in 1937 or later, 12% of the others). Younger doctors were also more likely to think that an elderly person adjusted better to widowhood if their spouse had died at home (79% of them, 65% of the older doctors thought this), but fewer of them thought it was always necessary to see a deceased person before signing the death certificate if the person died expectedly at home and the doctor had seen them a short while beforehand. (The proportions who thought this necessary were 59% of those born in 1937 or later, 75% of the others.)

There was no difference with the age of the doctor in the proportions who said they enjoyed looking after older people of pensionable age either more or less than younger people. Altogether 26% said they enjoyed caring for older people more, 12% less, and 61% that it made no difference (1% made other comments). Younger doctors were more likely than older ones to feel they were able to give enough time to recently widowed people: the proportions were 58% and 40%. And, as we showed earlier, they had seen more of their elderly widowed patients since their bereavement.

A final difference between the doctors of different ages was in their training: the proportion who had had a trainee year in general practice or been through a recognized vocational training scheme rose from 18% of those born before 1927 to 32% of those born in 1937 or later. What other differences were there associated with their training?

Training

Doctors were asked if they had had any specific training for general practice after qualifying. *Table 52* shows the types of training that were listed together with their replies. Several doctors indicated that they had had more than one type of training so for further analyses

Table 52   Specific training for general practice

	All types
	%
Recognized vocational training scheme	7
Training year in general practice	16
Assistantship in general practice	41
Self-organized vocational training scheme	10
Other training	1
No specific training	36
Number of doctors (= 100%)	179

Table 53   Training and types of area and practice

	Specific training for general practice			All general practitioners
	Ex-trainees	Ex-assistants	None	
Single-handed:	%	%	%	%
Yes	10	26	22	20
No	90	74	78	80
Has group practice allowance:	%	%	%	%
Yes	75	58	74	69
No	25	42	26	31
Type of area:	%	%	%	%
Designated	5	16	15	12
Open	35	44	54	47
Intermediate	45 } 60	34 } 40	19 } 31	31
Restricted	15	6	12	10
Uses deputizing services:	%	%	%	%
Regularly	27	29	46	35
Occasionally	20	25	11	17
Never	53	46	43	48
Described home help service for elderly patients in their area as:	%	%	%	%
Adequate	71	52	49	55
Rather inadequate	24	41	48	40
Very inadequate	5	7	3	5
Number of general practitioners (=·100%)	41	61	63	177

three main groups were considered: those with either a recognized vocational training scheme or a trainee year in general practice (the ex-trainees, amounting to 23%), those without either of these but who had had an assistantship (the ex-assistants amounting to 35%), and those with no specific training, 36%. The other 6% with various other types of training have been ignored in these comparisons.

While younger doctors were more likely to be ex-trainees, more of the older doctors were ex-assistants: 39% of those born before 1937 compared with 25% of the younger ones. Associated with the age differences, the ex-trainees were least likely to be in a single-handed practice while a comparatively small proportion of the ex-assistants had a group practice allowance. The figures are in *Table 53*. The ex-trainees were the ones least likely to be working in designated or open areas and the ones without any training were the ones most likely to do so. Possibly associated with this, those without any training were most likely to use a deputizing service regularly, while the ex-trainees were the ones most often in areas where they felt the home help service for the elderly was adequate. Training may benefit the individual doctors by enabling them to obtain work in more attractive areas but, from the point of view of the community, if it is an advantage to have a doctor with additional training, the less attractive areas are at a disadvantage. This can be seen as a further demonstration of Hart's inverse care law: 'the availability of good medical care tends to vary inversely with the need for it in the population served' (Hart 1971).

In this study, unlike the one in 1977 (Cartwright and Anderson 1981), training was unrelated to membership of the Royal College of General Practitioners, but on neither study was there any relationship between training and the doctors' estimates of the proportion of consultations that were trivial, inappropriate, or unnecessary or whether they felt it was appropriate for people to seek help from their general practitioner for problems in their family lives. In this study training did not appear to affect doctors' views on the frequency with which relatives of elderly people shirk their responsibilities nor their opinions about the care and supervision that general practitioners should give to the elderly bereaved.

Similar proportions of the three groups throught that elderly patients who had been widowed should be visited at home and that elderly bereaved patients should generally be given some supervision by their general practitioner for a while. But their views on two aspects of appropriate practice did vary significantly with training: ex-assistants were the ones most likely to think that elderly people who had recently been widowed should always or generally be offered a sedative — 68% of them thought this, 44% of the others. Possibly ex-assistants are more likely to express the most common viewpoint if they are influenced by the practices of the doctors they work with initially. In contrast, and in the opposite direction to that expected from the age variations, those with no specific training were the ones least likely to say the doctor should always see the body before signing the death certificate: 60% of them held this view, 78% of the others. It is hoped that further training might make doctors more aware of the emotional needs of patients, as opposed to their legal and clinical responsibilities. Over that point there is indication of some success.

Turning to the views and experiences of the widowed there were no differences between the three training groups in the proportion of the widowed who had had a home visit since their bereavement, in the proportion who had discussed their spouse's illness and impending death with a general practitioner, nor in their views of their doctor as being friendly or businesslike, easy to talk to, or having time to discuss things. Of the six criteria we have examined one showed a significant difference at the 5% level: doctors without any training were the ones most often felt to be 'very sympathetic'; 80% of their patients described them in this way compared with 64% of the patients with doctors who were ex-trainees or ex-assistants.

Types of practice

'People's relationships with and opinions about their doctors vary remarkably little with the number of doctors in the practice.' This conclusion from a study in 1964 (Cartwright 1967 : 150), endorsed in 1977 (Cartwright and Anderson 1981), is further substantiated on this study. From the viewpoint of the widowed there was no indication that they found doctors more or less sympathetic or easy to talk to if they worked single-handed or in a small or large group. The number of doctors in a practice did not even relate to the proportion of widowed who had seen *their own doctor* since their bereavement.

Neither was there any variation with the number of doctors in a practice in the general practitioners' attitudes – over trivial consultations, the appropriateness of consultation for family problems, the care that should be given to the elderly bereaved, and the frequency with which relatives avoid their responsibilities.

However, in the way they organized their practices there was a clear difference in both the 1977 study (Cartwright and Anderson 1981) and the present one: the proportion using a deputizing service was considerably higher among the single-handed than among the others – 75% against 44%. Other things related to the use of a deputizing service are considered next.

General practitioners who used a deputizing service regularly were also less likely to regard it as appropriate for patients to consult them about problems in their family lives: 63% of them did so compared with 85% of those who used one occasionally or never. From the point of view of the widowed, general practitioners using a deputizing service regularly were less often felt to have time to discuss things: 23% of the widowed with such a doctor felt this compared with 10% of the others. There was also some suggestion that the widowed had fewer home visits from any doctor if their general practitioner used a deputizing service: the average number of home visits reported since the death of their spouse was 0.71 if the doctor used such a service, 1.27 if he or she did not — but this last difference did not quite reach the 5% level of statistical significance.

Discussion

Probably the most disconcerting finding from this chapter is that general practitioners were apparently unaware of a sizeable proportion of the prescribed drugs that their elderly widowed patients were taking. And since this finding is supported by another study with a quite different approach and method, it is one that should be pursued. What are the reasons for it, and the implications?

The disparity between the doctors' perceptions and those of the widowed were often striking. Over loneliness and suitability of housing agreement was no better than it might have been by chance. Does this matter? If doctors are alert to the severely depressed, the social isolate, and the housebound, it may not be important from a clinical viewpoint or that of the community as a whole that they are unaware of the minor depressions, the lonely, and those who retain some mobility by struggling on to buses or up and down the stairs in their home. But from this study there is evidence that doctors may not be aware of treatable disability among their elderly patients even if they have seen the patients fairly recently, and they sometimes appear to be ignorant of the degree of immobility experienced by the elderly widowed.

What can be done to improve things? There is some evidence that older doctors are somewhat less sensitive to their patients' needs but it is not possible to tell whether their eventual retirement will improve things or whether the currently middle-aged will in their turn become less sympathetic as they grow older.

For full evaluation of the present vocational training programme we need to wait until it has been established for a longer time, since some of the 'ex-trainees' in our study may have undertaken their trainee year sometime ago when vocational training was in the early stages of development and the importance of pastoral care was not emphasized as much as it is in current schemes. But to date the evidence is hardly encouraging. There is no indication that doctors who have had experience as trainees have a generally wider concept of their role, and they are as likely as other doctors to regard a sizeable proportion of their consultations as trivial, unnecessary, or inappropriate. There is mounting evidence that doctors' estimates of the proportion of their consultations that are 'trivial' are strongly related to a number of other attitudes to their work. The outlook of those doctors who perceive relatives as often shirking their responsibilities, regard family problems as inappropriate topics for consultation, do not think they should visit their elderly patients who have been bereaved, categorize a high proportion of their consultations as trivial, and make regular use of deputizing services, is one of the more depressing aspects of general practice − which neither time, training, nor an increase in partnerships shows signs of changing.

7 Emotional adjustment, loneliness, and their concomitants

The death of a spouse not only means adjustment to a new, and in many ways a less well-defined, role but also having to cope with a painful emotional state. Indeed the death of a spouse probably has a greater impact on people in terms of their ability to adjust than any other event in their lives (Holmes and Rahe 1967). Marriage leads to some change in self-identity and the ending of marriage often impels a dramatic identity reformulation (Lopata 1973). Sometimes the strains are so great that bereavement in the elderly may lead to mental illness (Kay, Roth, and Hopkins 1955, and Parkes 1964).

So in this chapter we explore some of the factors that may relate to adaptation. We start by describing reactions to grief, go on to discuss various possible indicators of adjustment, and develop an adjustment scale. We then consider the concept of loneliness and how this relates to adjustment, after which we describe the ways in which adjustment and loneliness vary with various characteristics of the widowed, the circumstances of the death, and the marital relationship.

Reactions to bereavement

The main components, or stages, of grief have been described by Bowlby (1960) and Parkes (1972). The most common ones appear to be shock, often resulting in feelings of numbness and an inability to cry, perhaps accompanied by denial, which may lead to hallucinations involving the deceased; intense grief involving searching for the deceased; guilt, anxiety, leading to suicidal thoughts, and aggression — for example against doctors for not preventing the death or against the deceased for deserting them; depression and apathy; and finally re-integration. Some examples of these feelings have already been presented. Components can also be seen in the following statements:

'I couldn't cry. It was a fortnight or three weeks before I really cried. I went upstairs and found a birthday card to me in his drawer. My birthday's in January, he'd written it ready.'

'I've been so depressed I couldn't come in the house. . . . I still can't go to the cemetery, I start crying. The neighbours are so good. I cry and cry. I still see him everywhere. For four months I've done nothing. I dream as well.'

'You often think "I've got so many sleeping pills I would be better off out of it".'

A widow who felt guilty because she had not helped her husband more said 'I always feel that guilt'. One result was that she continually washed herself:

'I have too many baths now, I never used to have many baths in the other place.'

We asked our interviewers to assess whether the widows and widowers they talked to had finished grieving, were still grieving, or had not grieved. One in twenty of the widowed were thought to fall in this last category. One of these, a widow, had commented:

'I haven't been able to cry. I haven't cried yet. I wish I could − that's the trouble.'

At the other end of the scale a quarter were thought by the inter-viewers to have finished grieving, leaving seven-tenths who were still grieving (3% 'overwhelmingly', 28% 'some', and 38% 'a little'). The widowed who said they had come to terms with the death were much more likely than others to be assessed as having finished grieving, 96% in comparison with 63%. Also, those who were reported to have finished grieving were more likely than others to have said they wished to continue their lives in the same way, 86% in comparison with 72%. But of course these statements will have been taken into account by the interviewers in making the assessments. Parkes (1965) argues that the widowed cannot avoid grief − they can only postpone it and post-ponement may lead to greater emotional disturbance later on.

The familiars were asked a rather different question — whether they felt the widowed were predominantly living either in the past, or present, or whether they were in the process of adapting to a new life — a question we felt it was inappropriate to ask the widowed themselves. Twenty per cent of familiars said that the widow or widower was living in the past predominantly, 32% said he or she was in the process of adapting from an old to a new life, and 48% said he or she was living in the present predominantly.

We also asked familiars whether they thought the widow or widower was happy or not. Fifty-six per cent were said to be either very or fairly happy, 32% neither happy nor unhappy, 8% fairly unhappy, and 3% very unhappy. One per cent made other comments. The following types of comments were made by familiars of the widowed described as 'very unhappy':

'She's not really getting any better. She's not facing up to reality. She's depressed and has bad nights.'

'She's very unhappy and very unstable. She's very demanding — crazy really. . . . She's as highly depressed as you can get I think. I don't see her as a widow, I see her as someone with great mental trouble. . . . She drinks a lot of whisky and takes pills. I don't know what they are. She was found on the floor the other day because she'd mixed the alcohol and pills. She woke up in —— [hospital], and she was really rather proud of that. She teases life. She's made her will and set the whole scene for the widow to die. I don't think she's in charge of herself.'

'She says she wishes she could die and be with —— [deceased].'

'He's almost in limbo. I think he has put himself into a year's mourning. He's so forgetful — I can't help the mental problem.'

'Being deaf is a difficulty. She finds it hard to make friends.'

These give some idea of the intensity of problems faced by some of the widowed, but most of them were seen by the person who knew them best to be adapting to their new life, and few were felt to be deeply unhappy. What indication of their adjustment did we get from the widows and widowers themselves?

Indicators of adjustment

We asked the widowed a number of questions related to adjustment and in this section we give their responses to these in both statistical and illustrative terms, and then go on to show how their responses to the different questions were related.

In a direct question about adjustment we asked the widowed whether they felt they had come to terms with the death of their husband or wife. Seventy-one per cent felt they had done so, but 29% said they had not, including 9% who thought they would never do so. Most of the others thought they would do so eventually but were uncertain how long it would take.

While the majority responded positively about coming to terms with the death almost two-thirds of them, 66%, said they were unable to look forward to things in the same way as they did before the death:[1]

'There is a sense of loss when you think "we should have been doing this together".'

'I feel dead inside. I've no interest in life. What I do I push myself to do.'

'I used to look forward to going out those nights when the girls came up [to whist drives], now it doesn't matter to me.'

Twenty-three per cent felt they would be able to look forward to things later on, while 15% thought they would never be able to do so, and 28% were uncertain. Even among those who could look forward now, half (that is one in six of all the widowed) said there had been a time after the death when they could not do so. For most of them, three-quarters, this period lasted less than three months.

Another question about their current feelings asked the widowed whether they ever felt apart or remote, even among friends.[2] Over a quarter, 28%, said they did:

'When you're on your own you're an outsider.'

'You feel the odd one out. You feel on your own when you've always been out together.'

'[with] couples you feel you're intruding.'

'You're not included in the conversation, you're pushed to one side.'

Widows and widowers were asked to describe the way things were going for them.[3] Most, 90%, said things were going reasonably for

---

[1] 'Do you find now that you can look forward to things in the same way you used to before —— died?'

[2] Adapted from Parkes (1979).

[3] The actual questions are quoted in full on p. 70.

them these days, while 6% said they were not going very well, and 3% said they were not going at all well. This may reflect low aspirations and expectations. Hunt (1978) found that old people expressed more satisfaction with their lives than younger people. It is possible that some responses reflect a degree of resignation. Three-quarters of the widowed said they wished their lives to continue in much the same way, a fifth wanted to change some parts of it, and 3% to change many parts of it.[3] Among the minority who were looking for a change, a desire to move, to start going out, and to make new friends, were among the things mentioned. For example:

'To get out. I wish I could have more company.'

'Moving and to get out on my own.'

'At first I used to cry all day — I never stopped. Now I think about moving and getting a job and somehow starting again.'

'To be able to get about and try to mix with people. You see I've never been a mixer but I wish I could now. If I could find a few friends. . . . As it is now I can't go very far and people I know can get about, you lag behind. I could have gone away with my daughter but I'm frightened of spoiling their holiday. They're good walkers.'

A desire to re-marry was also expressed:

'If I could find a widow to come and share my house.'

Not all wanted to make a fresh start however. One said she wanted 'it to end soon' and seemed to be looking forward only to her own death. Another simply said:

'I'd like to go back to having my wife with me again.'

How did these different indicators of adjustment relate to each other? *Table 54* shows the five questions listed in order of the proportion giving a response indicating adjustment, and the significance of the association between the answers. All the associations, except that between 'things going reasonably well' and 'not feeling remote among friends' were highly significant. We decided to combine them together into a crude adjustment scale from nought to five, scoring one for each of the questions to which they gave an answer indicating adjustment. We did this to simplify the presentation of the results and because the combination was likely to be more sensitive than the

Table 54   The different indicators of adjustment and the significance of the association between them

	Percentage 'adjusted'	Association				
		Things going reasonably well	Wants to continue in same way	Has come to terms with death	Does not feel remote among friends	Able to look forward
Things going reasonably well	90%	–				
Wants to continue in same way	75%	**	–			
Has come to terms with death	71%	**	*	–		
Does not feel remote among friends	70%	0	*	*	–	
Able to look forward	32%	*	*	**	**	–

* p < .01
** p < .001
0 p > .10

response to a single question. The average score was 3.4 and the distribution is shown in *Table 55*.

Before considering the personal characteristics and social circumstances associated with adjustment, we look at the rather different concept of loneliness and consider first whether and how this is related to our index of adjustment. We will then be able to see whether the concomitants of loneliness and adjustment are similar.

Loneliness

The most common problem identified by the widowed in our study was loneliness: 33% gave this reply to a question on particular problems in their life now.[4] Tunstall (1966) found that the widowed generally had a greater chance of being lonely than married or single old people. This loneliness may lead to feelings of social isolation, boredom, and vulnerability. Townsend (1957) found that the loss of a loved person is more important than social isolation in explaining the loneliness of old people. The widowed may feel lonely because they are no longer the object of a spouse's love and attention, rather than because of an isolating life style and loss of activities engaged in as

[4] 'Thinking about your life now – is there anything that you feel is a particular problem?'

Table 55 Distribution on adjustment scale

	%
Score:	
0	2
1	5
2	17
3	25
4	29
5	22
Average	3.4
Number of widowed (= 100%)	342

a couple. The loss of their intimate partner − and the consequent gap left − was often felt acutely by the widowed in the present study:

'You come in from the garden and you have to get your own meals, you go to bed and there's no one to talk to.'

'I feel I can't cope. I'm lonely. I miss his companionship. I'm like somebody who has lost a limb. I go up to the cemetery on my own with flowers, I saw a man and wife there and I had a bout of crying. I don't know what's wrong with me.'

'I sometimes have a feeling of emptiness seeing other women with their hubbys. I went to a party and I had to come home − they all wondered what was wrong. It wasn't like me. I'm usually the life and soul of the party.'

Lopata (1973) found half the widows in her sample regarded loneliness as their most serious difficulty. Similarly in the present study, half the widowed found loneliness to be a problem. A quarter said it was a big problem while a fifth thought they would get over it soon − the rest made other comments:

'Loneliness − [crying] − I could put up with it better if I knew it was just a week or two, but it's forever.'

'When people are here I'm allright but when I'm on my own I start howling.'

Our index of adjustment was clearly related to feelings of loneliness: the average on the adjustment scale fell from 3.9 for those who did not

feel loneliness was a problem to 2.6 for those who found it a big problem. (It was 3.2 for the intermediate group who thought they would
get over their loneliness fairly soon or who made other comments.)

So is the expression of loneliness simply one aspect of adjustment?
Glick, Weiss, and Parkes (1974) found loneliness did not fade with
time, dropping comparatively little during the year following
bereavement. In the following sections we see whether the same
factors are associated with loneliness and poor adjustment.

Sex and age

Earlier we showed that widows and widowers did not differ in their
attitudes to their new domestic tasks although the nature of the tasks
was rather different. Neither did they differ in their acceptance of
living alone, and similar proportions of widows and widowers
reported problems of loneliness. But the widowers had a higher
adjustment score than the widows: 3.7 compared with 3.2. This suggests that widows were either finding it more difficult to adjust
emotionally to their new role, or they were more prepared to recognize and talk about the difficulty.

It has generally been found that women adjust to bereavement
worse than men (Clayton, Desmarais, and Winokur 1968; Parkes
1972). Possibly this is because being a wife is a more important part of
self-identity than is being a husband. Lopata (1971) suggested that
because they live in a male-dominated society and have been social-
ized into restricted roles, they face greater difficulties developing
social activities following widowhood. Also a wife's role is husband-
centred, and she is more often dependent on him for money, status,
and company than he is on her. Thus Parkes (1972) has said that loss
of a husband is the commonest type of relationship dissolution to give
rise to psychological difficulties. However, the difficulties for elderly
widowers too should not be underestimated. They have not only experienced the disruptions of retirement but, as they are held to be less
expressive than women, it may sometimes be more difficult for them
to work through their grief. One in five of the widowers cried during
the interview; two out of five of the widows.

Younger widows and widowers were more likely to find loneliness a
problem and to have more problems in adjustment. The figures are in
Table 56. Lopata (1971) suggested that younger widows feel their
widowhood more acutely as they have been bereaved before their

Table 56   Variations in loneliness and adjustment with age

	Age of widow or widower		
	Under 60	60–69	70 or more
Loneliness:	%	%	%
A big problem	52	31	19
Intermediate	24	25	26
No problem	24	44	55
Average adjustment score	2.6	3.2	3.6
Number of widowed (= 100%)	25	117	208

friends. She suggests that this may not only lead to social isolation in a society orientated towards couples, but they are now viewed as threats to husbands, by virtue of their availability. Widowers, of course, may pose a similar threat to friends' wives. Blau (1961 and 1973), too, has suggested that the prevalence of widowhood among one's age/sex peers is extremely important. Cumming and Henry (1961) refer to the 'society of widows' open to elderly women, a society not available for the young widow who is less likely to have contemporaries who have been widowed. Older age groups may also adjust better because they may more readily accept death if they feel they have fulfilled their lives. In addition, Kalish (1976) and Kalish and Reynolds (1976) found that older people talk and think more about death than younger people.

Class and money

Lopata (1973) found that middle-class, more highly-educated widows adjusted less well than others. She argues that these widows, during marriage, place more emphasis on their role as wife, concentrating their activities around their husbands, sharing tasks and activities with them, in contrast to those in the lower social classes. She further argued that less well educated women in the lower social classes place more significance on motherhood, whilst the more educated middle-class women regard marriage and being a wife as a major event in their lives. And as we mentioned earlier in Chapter 4, Rainwater (1965) found similar social-class differences. Consequently, widow-hood might be expected to lead to a more dramatic identity crisis in

Table 57   Variations in adjustment and loneliness with money problems

	Average adjustment score	Proportion finding loneliness:		Number of widowed (= 100%)
		A big problem	No problem	
Money a problem:				
Yes	2.9	36%	34%	101
No	3.6	22%	55%	238
Financially now:				
No worse off	3.6	17%	57%	134
A little worse off	3.7	22%	57%	68
A moderate amount worse off	3.1	36%	47%	60
A great deal worse off	2.9	37%	24%	56
*Goes short of something they need:**				
Yes	2.7	33%	30%	27
No	3.4	31%	45%	134
Financial position sorted out:				
Yes	3.5	25%	50%	281
No	2.9	28%	44%	65

* Those who said they were no worse off have been excluded because they were not asked this question.

middle-class people. However, although the expected relationship between task division before death and social class was partly supported by the present study, we found no class differences in either adjustment or loneliness. This failure to find a relationship with social class may be the result of confounding associations: both loneliness and adjustment were related to money problems and these were more common among the working class than the middle class.

The relationship between money difficulties and adjustment and loneliness are shown in *Table 57*. The index of adjustment related to all the questions about money problems, while loneliness was more often reported by those who found money a problem, and varied with the extent to which the widowed saw themselves as being worse off financially since the death of their spouse. However loneliness, unlike adjustment, did not seem to be aggravated by delay in getting their financial position sorted out.

A cross-analysis by social class and by those finding money a problem still revealed no class differences in either adjustment or loneliness, so our findings on this do not support those of Lopata (1973).

One way in which money difficulties may accentuate problems of loneliness and difficulties in adjustment is by inhibiting widows and widowers from developing meaningful activities and, as we will show next, feelings about the lack of such activities were clearly related to our index of adjustment and to feelings of loneliness.

Activities

It may seem surprising at first that the widowed who were working were no more or less likely to have difficulties in adjusting or to have problems of loneliness. But of course it was the younger ones who were more likely to have a job (44% of those under sixty-five were working, 10% of the older widowed) and as we have just seen it was the younger widows and widowers who were more likely to have difficulties on both these scores.

Those who found it difficult to occupy themselves[5] were less likely to have a high adjustment score as were those who had given up doing something since their spouse died (see *Table 58*). In addition loneliness was more often a problem among those who had difficulties in occupying themselves but the differences in loneliness with stopping certain activities did not reach a level of statistical significance. Quite a number had stopped doing things since their spouse's death because of increasing age and infirmity but for others it was a cut back in their social life. One had stopped 'going out for drinks or visiting' and another had 'stopped going to the theatre regularly – we used to go every fortnight'. Yet others seemed to take less pride in their home: 'I don't polish my furniture like I used to.'

The problem was not just having something to do – but having something they enjoyed. Those who had additional household tasks to do since their spouse died scored no better or worse on our adjustment scale than those who did not, but those who liked their new tasks had an average score of 3.7, compared with 3.0 for those who said they disliked them or had 'mixed feelings' about them.

[5] Those working full-time were not asked this question about difficulty in occupying themselves during the day.

Table 58   Variations in adjustment and loneliness with activities

	Average adjustment score	Proportion finding loneliness:		Number of widowed (= 100%)
		A big problem	No problem	
Finds it difficult to occupy self during the day: *				
Frequently	2.3	59%	16%	32
Occasionally	2.8	62%	16%	37
Never	3.6	16%	59%	252
Finds it difficult to occupy self in the evenings:				
Frequently	2.5	68%	8%	48
Occasionally	3.0	39%	24%	62
Never	3.7	13%	64%	231
Would like to do something else if it could be arranged:				
Yes	3.0	37%	33%	57
No	3.5	23%	52%	285
Has stopped doing something since bereaved:				
Yes	2.8	34%	40%	68
No	3.5	24%	51%	279

* Those working full-time were not asked the question about difficulty in occupying themselves during the day.

Having a dog, a cat, or any other type of pet did not seem to help adjustment, and those with some sort of pet were no less lonely than those without one. But those who had a dog were less likely to find loneliness a problem, 36% compared with 54%, although the proportion finding loneliness a big problem was similar for dog owners and those without one.

When asked if there was anything else they would like to do during the day or evening if this could be arranged 16% said there was. More of the younger widowed, under 65, said this: 29% compared with

14% of those aged 65 or more. Going to clubs, visiting people or having visitors, and driving a car were among the things mentioned. Lack of friends or close relatives, reluctance to impose themselves on others, fear of travelling alone late at night, and no access to a car were among the reasons given for not doing these things:

'I don't like encroaching on their time.'

'I don't know anyone who would come.'

'The buses are too late, it's getting home.'

'I haven't got a car.'

Less than a fifth, 14%, of the widowed had a car now, and 8% said another person in the same household had a car. Those living with others were more likely to have, or have access to, a car, 51% in comparison with 15%. A quarter of all the widowed had been deprived of access to a car as a result of their spouse's death. Some were finding that a problem:

'Of course I can't drive now, that's a big loss. She was my public relations man.'

So the activities of a sizeable minority had been cut back because of lack of transport and this meant a reduction in outings and curtailed the things they had to look forward to. Holidays too are objects of pleasurable anticipation. As we saw earlier, in Chapter 4, holidays were mentioned more often than anything else as something the widowed would like to have if they had a bit more money to spend. And when asked whether they expected to have a holiday in the next year or so, two-fifths said no and two-fifths of these, 15% of all widowed, said they would like one. The main reasons for not expecting to go on holiday were expense and not having anyone to go with.

Further links between money and activities are illustrated by the fact that those who found money a problem were more likely to have given up some activity since their spouse died − 29% of them had done so compared with 16% of those who did not find money a problem − and 31% of those finding money a problem also had difficulties occupying themselves during the day against 17% of the others.

What part did and could clubs and organizations play in helping the elderly widowed people to meet and make friends?

Clubs and organizations

Less than half, 42%, of the widowed went to clubs, or societies, or day centres. Old people's clubs (including pensioners, Darby and Joan, and retirement clubs) were the ones most often mentioned, by 13% of all the widowed, then church or religious groups by 7%, women's institutes or guilds by 6%, and working men's clubs by 5%. Some described how going to clubs and being with people had helped them:

'Loneliness could be a major problem but I keep myself busy with organizations, so that does help a bit. I think it's better if you're in some kind of organization where you can meet people — I think that's essential.'

'When I am amongst people all the time I can forget myself and when I am not with them then I try to do things and not think.'

But loneliness was just as likely to be a problem for those going to clubs as for those who did not. It may of course be that being lonely was sometimes a reason for going to clubs. The club attenders and non-attenders had similar scores on our adjustment scale but the few, 6% of all the widowed, who were not going to any clubs but said they would like to do so had a low average score, 2.5. Possibly some adaptation to widowhood is necessary before people are prepared to make the effort to be sociable in that sort of way. And some were resistant to the idea of going to clubs. The daughter of one widow described how she had tried to persuade her mother to join an old people's club:

'I suggested she tried to join the over sixties but she snapped "I couldn't do anything like that". I said she should give it a try but she could never mix, even when she was young. But then she always went with Dad. Now she won't make the effort. A social worker came and when I asked her how she got on she said she had a good talk. She mentioned the over sixties club and the social worker said she could understand how my mother felt because she would be the same if it was her. I didn't think that was the right thing for her to have said do you? I'll give it the twelve months and see the vicar to see if he can get her to join.'

The widow said she could not think of anything that could be done to help her with the problem of loneliness:

'I say to my daughter "Look I can't change. I've always been like this, quiet like." I've always been quiet. Even when I'm out I can't find anything to talk about.'

Joining in activities does not always help those who find communicating with others difficult. Another widow said:

'I don't make friends easily. But if anyone wants to make friends with me I'm quite willing.'

Existing clubs were not always seen as appropriate, nor was it always possible to join in activities, as the following comments indicate:

'They asked me to join. I asked what they did and they said "We're going to a disco." I didn't fancy that.'

'I know the answer is to keep busy, but I get so tired I can't hop about like I used to. My mind is active but my body will not work so well these days.'

The few, 6%, who did not go to any clubs but said they would like to do so were asked why they did not go. Sometimes they had 'not got round to it yet' — 'I'm too damned lazy to get ready to go out.' Other reasons were distance, 'it's too far to get to', transport problems, and no clubs in their area. Further difficulties were:

'I believe you have to have someone to sponsor you to get into them. I don't know any old people so I don't know how to go about it.'

'They are all full up and you have to wait twelve months. I might be gone then — it's ridiculous.'

We asked the widowed if they thought it might help to meet other people who had lost their husbands or wives. Almost half, 47%, said yes. Those who said loneliness was a problem were more likely to say they thought it might help, 50% compared with 39% of those for whom loneliness was not a problem. In fact there is an organization, Cruse, which aims to help the widowed mainly by mutual discussion. Sixteen per cent of the widowed said they knew such an organization existed,[6] only 1% knew its name. Those who did not know of such an organization were asked if they thought it would be a good idea to have such an organization: 42% were in favour, 32% did not think it a good idea, 26% were uncertain or made other comments. Several of

[6] 'Do you think it might help to meet other people who have lost their husbands or wives or not?'. 'Do you know if there is any organization that arranges that?'.

those who did not think it was a good idea indicated that they were well supported by family and friends, although no significant differences emerged with our indices of family support:

'I've got the family. I'm not a mixer, it wouldn't be for me.'

'You usually know enough people in your own circle.'

'I'd rather be on my own, everyone's friendly round here.'

Others said they did not want to hear about other people's problems:

'I was talking to a woman the other day who had lost her husband and she made me feel very depressed, talking about her family. I didn't say anything to her but I thought I don't want to hear your problems I've got enough of my own.'

'I had a friend who came round here and drank three schooners of my sherry. All he did was sit and talk about his wife and cry. I felt a damned sight worse when he left.'

Only one widow in our study had actually been in contact with Cruse and she had not joined them although she said she might do so in the future.

Beliefs and philosophies

Nearly half, 47%, of the widowed said they had a belief, philosophy, or practice which they felt had helped them to adjust to or accept their widowhood. A much higher proportion, 96%, said they had a religion. Most, 65%, described themselves as Church of England, 19% as 'other Protestant', 10% as Catholic, while 4% said they had no religion. The proportion who felt their beliefs or philosophy had been helpful to them was highest, 61%, among the Catholics; 56% among the 'other Protestants', and 43% among the Church of England. A third of the small group with no religion felt they had a philosophy which had been of help to them.

The belief that they would join their spouses in the future gave some of the widowed hope:

'When my time comes I believe that I shall go to join my husband. Sometimes when I'm feeling down, I have a lovely photo of him, I get it out and say to him "Help me". I'm sure he does in some way. I think to myself "Don't give way because I'm going to see him again one day".'

'I believe I shall join him before long. It gives me comfort. We had a good life together.'

Other comments about their beliefs or philosophies were:

'My Christian belief. Without that I think I would have gone under.'

'I believe that when Gabriel puts his number on your balloon you'll go. Drink for today for tomorrow you may be gone.'

'I'm a humanist − I believe in having the most out of life while I'm here.'

'My philosophy is to bounce back. I've had some hard knocks. I was left with four children when I was younger.'

Those who felt they had a helpful philosophy, however, had a similar score on our adjustment scale to those without one and there was no difference in the extent of loneliness reported by the two groups. There was no difference between widows and widowers in the proportion reporting a belief, philosophy, or practice which had helped them to adjust.

Health

Not surprisingly those in poor health experienced more difficulties in adjustment. The average adjustment score rose from 2.8 for those who described their health for their age as poor to 3.6 for those who rated it as excellent. There was also a clear link between loneliness and ill health: the proportion who found loneliness a problem fell from 69% of those in poor health to 40% of those who rated their health as excellent.

Difficulties in getting around also seemed to make adjustment more difficult. Those with mobility problems[7] had an average adjustment score of 3.2 compared with 3.5 without such problems, but similar proportions of the mobile and immobile reported problems with loneliness. In a later chapter we shall see whether those experiencing difficulties in getting around had more or less contact with relatives and friends.

Turning to specific symptoms, the few who reported none at all out of a list of 15,[8] had a high average adjustment score of 4.2, while

[7] Had difficulties with or could not do on own − use public transport, go out, go up and down stairs, get in and out of bath.
[8] For list see p. 97, *Table 34.*

Table 59   Loneliness and symptoms associated with it

	Widowed finding loneliness:		
	A big problem	Intermediate	No problem
Proportion reporting:			
Headaches	39%	25%	21%
Sleeplessness	72%	48%	39%
Corns, bunions or trouble with feet	41%	34%	26%
Nerves or depression	69%	51%	30%
Loss of appetite	30%	16%	8%
Number of widowed (= 100%)	88	73	168

symptoms associated with a low score were loss of appetite (2.6), irritability (2.8), nerves and depression (2.8), sleeplessness (3.0), and headaches (3.0). Earlier we showed that loss of appetite, nerves or depression, and sleeplessness were the symptoms which were most often said to develop or become worse after their spouse's death. In addition, loss of appetite, nerves or depression, sleeplessness, headaches, but also trouble with feet, were related to loneliness, as can be seen from *Table 59*. Possibly the widowed with foot problems were less able, or less inclined, to go and see their relatives and friends.

Circumstances of death

Several factors which might affect adjustment have been suggested in previous chapters: those involved in the long-term caring of the deceased may find it more difficult to adjust because they have now lost their main occupation; on the other hand the length of the terminal illness may enable survivors to work through many of their feelings regarding the loss prior to the actual death. Glick, Weiss, and Parkes (1974) found anticipation of the death to be one of the most important determinants of recovery, and some of the widowed on this study commented that knowledge of, leading to preparation for, the death would have lessened the shock for them.

We found no association between our index of adjustment and the length of time the spouse had been ill, the place of death, or whether or not the widow or widower had known their spouse was likely to die or described the death as expected. Nor was loneliness related to the length of illness, knowledge of the prognosis, or whether the death was expected or not. But those whose spouse had died at home were less likely to say that loneliness was a big problem for them than those whose husband or wife had died in hospital − 19% against 32%. We thought this might be related to attachment to their home. When those still living in the home they had shared with their spouse were asked, 'At the moment do you feel the memories associated with your present home make you want to move away or to stay?', the lonely were less likely to want to stay. This proportion rose from 71% of those who found loneliness a big problem to 85% of those who said it was no problem. But this did not vary significantly between those whose spouse had died at home or in hospital.

In contrast, the widowed person's *feelings* about what had happened appeared to be strongly related to their adjustment. Those who wished something had been done differently seemed to be finding it more difficult to adjust: their average score on our scale was 2.8 compared with 3.6 for those who did not express such a wish. Associated with this, those who were critical of the way their spouse had been looked after in hospital had a lower adjustment − 3.0, against 3.5 for those who described the way they had been looked after as 'very good'. There was no such relationship between adjustment and the widowed person's view of the way the general practitioner had looked after their spouse, but those who said their husband or wife had had no contact with a general practitioner in the last year of their lives had a relatively low score − 2.9 compared with 3.4 for the others. Wishing things had been done differently was also related to feelings of loneliness afterwards: 38% of those who felt unhappy about something that happened before the death said loneliness was a big problem, 22% of the others. Those who thought the care given to their spouse was inadequate may have had feelings of guilt which inhibited their adjustment and intensified their loneliness.

Nature of relationship

People who have had a good relationship with their husband or wife may feel a greater sense of deprivation when they are widowed than those who have had a poor relationship, but even without love marriage can give an emotional security which is lost at widowhood.

The intensity of grief does not necessarily vary with the intensity of love and may be even greater if feelings within the marriage were mixed (see Marris 1974). Those who were unhappily married may be more likely to harbour bitterness, resentment, and guilt and perhaps be less able to come to terms with their emotions. One widow, identified as one of those with multiple adjustment problems, said she had a bad relationship with her husband and now felt guilty as she felt she should have given him more care:

'I am missing him a lot. I always feel that guilt.'

She said he had been violent with her during their marriage, but felt that if she had known he was dying she would have treated him better:

'I was terribly frightened of him in the last six years. He knocked me around a lot. I feel I'm not a normal person. I've had a lot of bashing around.'

She did not think she would ever come to terms with the death:

'I don't think I'll ever conquer it. There's a big gap in me.'

The widowed who had had a poor relationship with their spouse may have felt some relief at their death. A different sort of relief may be felt by those whose spouse had been ill for some time, or had been in pain or suffering from distressing symptoms. We did not feel it was appropriate to ask the widowed directly about their feelings of relief, but we asked their familiars and our interviewers to make assessments about this. Thirty-six per cent of the widowed were said by their familiars to be relieved, and 38% of them were thought by our interviewers to have experienced some relief. These assessments were made completely independently as the interviewers who saw the widow or widower and made the assessment did not interview the familiar, who was always seen by a different interviewer. But there was a strong association between the two: 70% of those reported by the familiar to have experienced some relief were assessed by the interviewer to have done so, compared with 26% of those not regarded by the familiar as having a sense of relief. Interviewers thought that a third of all the widowed felt relief just because of the illness or need for care, but one in fifteen were thought by the interviewers to have felt relief at least partly because of the nature of their relationship. Most of the widowed, 89%, were thought by the interviewers to have had a 'good' or 'very good' relationship with their spouse, and those with a less

good relationship were more likely to have felt relief at their death —
83% were thought to have done so compared with 33% of the other
widowed. Feelings of relief did not, however, appear to be related to
adjustment, and indeed the situations which led to the relief may also
have resulted in feelings of guilt which might have inhibited adjustment. Some descriptions of the situations in which familiars perceived
relief were:

'It was definitely so in my auntie's case [relief]. It upset her to see
him like that [confused] because he had been a clever man.'

'I think it was [relief]. Mum realized it was getting to the point
where she couldn't cope, and he was so tired.'

'I think my aunt realized he had suffered. She also felt that if he
continued he was going to need more help.'

Although we did not ask the widowed directly about any feeling of
relief, a few mentioned it spontaneously. One widow who did so said:

'I think life is just opening up for me at last. It has taken fifty-three
years. I'm doing all the things he wouldn't let me do. I can play my
records and read a book in peace. I used to wonder why God was
letting me suffer. Now I have my reward.'

A widower who was now living with his nephew's widow said:

'I can look forward to things in a better way now. Dorothy and I
have had a lovely holiday in Ireland. We had a caravan, we've got a
good relationship, we've got a lot in common. . . . We (self and
deceased) never slept in the same room for thirty years and I had to
put a bar on my door to stop her wandering in and out. She used to
wander about. Well, there's Dorothy now.'

Relief may be a predominant feeling for those with unhappy marital
histories. Another type of relief may follow the end of a long period of
suffering for the deceased:

'Because he was ill so long I prayed he should die. The doctor said
he wasn't suffering but I knew he was in pain. You know when you
live with somone all those years how they are. That was worse than
anything.'

Also a number of the widowed mentioned the independence and
release from duties which accompany widowhood: 'I can do what I
like now'; 'my time's my own'.

162   Life After A Death

One hypothesis arising from our preliminary inquiries was that those widows and widowers whose life had centred around their spouse would find it more difficult to adjust than those who had led more independent lives. Two quotations illustrate this possibility:

'I would like to have gone first. I suppose that's selfish but it is too much of a heartbreak for me. We just lived for each other and didn't go out and make new friends and now there isn't time to make a new life. We relied on each other too much. I don't want it to go on as it is now. It is too much of a fight. I would like to find some way to change it. We had such a happy life and I have such happy memories but you can't re-live memories. They have gone. All that is left is an awful void and an emptiness. . . . I sometimes think that if I had my life over again I would try not to live such a narrow married life. We just lived for each other and in a way that is wrong. Whichever partner is left it makes it much harder to bear and to become stabilized again.'

In contrast, a widow in her late fifties who was working full-time said:

'We were close, but we had independent and mutual friends and social activities. . . . I wouldn't want to live with anyone else. I'm quite content. No one will ever take his place.'

We therefore asked familiars, 'Would you say ——— (widow/er's) life tended to be centred round his/her wife/husband or did he/she have independent activities of his/her own?'. Almost three-quarters, 73%, said the widowed person's life had centred mainly round the deceased, 24% said they had independent activities, and 3% made other comments. But this did not relate to our adjustment scale even though 92% of the widowed said to have independent activities wished to continue their lives in the same way, in comparison with 72% with none. However those with independent activities were less likely to find loneliness a problem: 38% of them described it as a problem compared with 60% of those whose life had centred round their spouse.

We also asked familiars if they could tell us anything else about the couple's relationship which might have affected the widow's or widower's ability to cope alone. Familiars sometimes replied either that the widow was dependent on the deceased or that they had both become dependent on each other:

'They never went anywhere without each other. She [widow] relied on him for every social contact. Mother doesn't like mixing at all.'

'She wasn't physically fit to cope on her own. She depended on him.'

'He [deceased] was always there and they always went out with each other.'

'She's so used to waiting on him hand and foot she's lost without him.'

Other comments indicated that the widow or widower was coping now because the couple's relationship involved some independence:

'They married late. She was always independent. She held down a good job for years and was very independent.'

'She's always been very independent. She'll get on and do things, so I think she can cope with most things.'

A question to the widowed, which gave some indication of their relationship with their spouse, asked when they missed their husband or wife most. Nearly a third, 30%, said it was all the time, but the most difficult times seemed to be evenings or night time − mentioned specifically by 46%; other times mentioned included meal times by 5%, mornings by 8%, and afternoons by 4%:

'It's not so bad during the day when you do your jobs and shopping. But it's when you come to sit down at night.'

'You can be in the middle of a crowd and it'll suddenly come over you, but definitely [it's] when I come in at night. When I've walked the dog and I put the key in the door, that's definitely not a nice feeling.'

Six, 2%, said they never missed their spouses. One widow who never missed her spouse now was critical of their previous relationship:

'We didn't talk much. He'd sit and look out of the window for hours. He never got up to bed until one o'clock and I liked to go to bed early. I couldn't sleep until he was in bed, I had to check if he'd left the fire on, or the TV.'

She said it was a relief to her when he died and added:

'When people stop me out shopping and talk about their dead husbands they get on my nerves.'

She lived alone now but said she was not lonely and nothing in her life was a particular problem. She could look forward to things and was content with her life now:

> 'I'm free to do as I like. To tell the truth, the week I spent with my son before the funeral, I felt better than I'd done for years. There were lots of things going on. We were busy with all the arrangements and buying clothes for the funeral.'

Another widow said she had a poor relationship with her husband and even regretted her marriage:

> 'Before I got married to him I used to have a social life. I used to visit the elderly sick, and I used to go to church, but after I got married all that stopped. I should have left him a fortnight after I'd married him. I was a lot worse off. He wouldn't buy me a pair of tights or an item of clothing.'

This widow said that her husband had been mentally confused in the year before his death, he had tried to strangle her and threatened to poison her. She added:

> 'Well I knew I couldn't carry on much longer with the life we had had. . . . You've no idea what a relief it was when it [the death] happened.'

When he died she said she was 'stone-faced', and that she could not believe it, she was so relieved:

> 'I slept the sleep of righteousness when I got home.'

Again, no feelings of loneliness or poor adjustment seemed to be experienced.

One widower who said he did not miss his spouse had been unable to sleep while his wife was alive as she would wander about at night. He was unable to go out with his wife since she was incontinent, and he gave up visiting people, going out socially and on holiday, and entertaining at home. He said their home smelt strongly of urine. He was not lonely although he lived alone, was content with his life, and was able to look forward to things.

A second widower who said he never missed his wife was also content and did not find loneliness a problem; he lived with his son. He simply commented:

> 'I've got my mate — my dog — and my son, so I've got plenty of

company. I've got my own friends, I can sit with them when I want a chatter and a pint. I go and have my beer — that's all I need.'

The remaining two, one widow and one widower, who never missed their spouses had both moved after the death. The widow lived with her son and the widower with his daughter. Both were content now and did not feel lonely. The widower commented that he and his wife had 'gone their own ways'.

Conclusion

Earlier we described how the transition to widowhood could happen suddenly without any warning, although, for older people, it was more often a culmination of a lengthy period of looking after an increasingly frail, disabled, and quite frequently confused spouse. In this chapter we have shown how the experience of losing a husband or wife varied with the nature of the relationship: from the devastation of losing the one person with whom the widow or widower had a close and loving relationship, to the relief of being freed from a difficult and burdensome oppression or the anxiety of caring for someone who was mentally confused or in pain.

We have shown that a wide range of factors appear to contribute to the emotional adjustment and to the loneliness of the widowed. But one of the problems in identifying associations between feelings about adjustment and attitudes to both past and present experiences is that one may colour the other. Those who have been able to make an adjustment may interpret the past rather differently from those who are still struggling to come to terms with their bereavement. So feelings about the past may be influenced by present perspectives rather than the other way round.

Our findings suggest that many of the circumstances of the death — its place, its expectedness, and the length of illness preceding it — did not have a direct relationship with adjustment. Neither did our measures of people's religion, beliefs, or philosophy.

Those who found it most difficult to adjust and were more likely to feel lonely were characterized by being female, comparatively young, in poor health, and having mobility problems. They also found it more difficult to occupy their time and more of them had financial problems, and earlier we showed that money problems also seemed to make it more difficult for the widowed to accept living alone. Another series of variables which seem likely to be important — contacts and relationships with relatives and friends — are examined in the next chapter.

8 Isolation and the role of relatives and friends

Two aspects of isolation have been identified in previous chapters: the practical one of living alone and the subjective one of loneliness. The two were clearly related, but although those who lived with others were less likely to find loneliness a problem, 34% in comparison with 56% who lived alone, a significant minority who were lonely still existed among those sharing a home. This is probably explained by feelings of emotional, rather than social isolation. We saw in the last chapter that the widowed who were described by their familiars as having had independent activities of their own, rather than a life which centred round their spouse, were less likely to find loneliness a problem. Those who were gregarious and had always had outside activities, friends, and visitors might continue to enjoy them, while those who had not led such an active life were probably unlikely to develop one upon widowhood. One widow, for example, said that now she often saw no one for two weeks at a time. Others commented:

'I've never been on my own [before]. We were two together, we never went out except together. He liked to go out for a drink but he never went out unless I came too. I was never indoors, hardly, on my own.'

'I don't think I'll ever conquer it. There's a big gap in me. We shared our friends, we didn't go our own ways. We were always together. . . . I'd know the wife since I was fourteen, we'd never been out without each other. As time goes on I seem to miss her more. I'm getting tense and nervous and quick tempered.'

'We both had such a sheltered life. We didn't go out drinking.'

Another widow told us that she had also been lonely with her marriage:

> 'My husband, at night, would sit and go to sleep. It wasn't like being with someone who was always on the go. I used to think if anyone tries to break in he wasn't able to help me, but when he was gone I really missed him. It used to upset me a bit when I'd turn to talk to him and he'd be asleep.'

So loneliness is not simply a function of living alone and no longer having a husband or wife. What part do relationships with relatives and friends play in this and in the adjustment of elderly widowed people to their new status? Before attempting to answer this, we look at the contacts the widows and widowers had with various relatives and friends.

Contacts with relatives and friends

In contrast to pre-industrial societies in which the different generations and branches of a family lived together, the focus of life within industrialized nations is on the nuclear family. Consequently, the elderly are more likely to live alone. In addition, increasing geographical mobility and the increasing proportions of women who work result in the family being less able to help elderly relatives. With smaller families there are also fewer sons and daughters to care for parents. So, the increasing problem of our society is that we have more old people who are growing older than ever before. Looking after them are a smaller number of family members.

On the other hand, Townsend's (1957) study indicated that the loss of the extended family has been exaggerated. Interaction with kin, particularly between older parents and their children, was found to be a frequent and important part of people's lives. Shanas and her colleagues (1968), comparing the situation of elderly people in the United States, Great Britain, and Denmark, further suggested that the aged are more strongly integrated into industrial society than is commonly assumed. These authors also argued that the loss of a marriage partner in old age tends to deepen the bond between remaining family members. Thus, research findings do not, on the whole, confirm the negative stereotype of old age that the Hendricks' (1978) found prevalent among the public, in which most elderly people are isolated from their families. What of the widowed in our sample?

Table 60   The widows' and widowers' supporters

	Person seen most often	Person most comfort	Person who gave most practical help
Relationship to widowed person:	%	%	%
Son	15	15	19
Daughter	26	32	32
Brother	3	1	1
Sister	4	5	5
Other male relative	2	2	3
Other female relative	5	9	7
Male friend	3	1	2
Female friend	22	12	11
People from more than one category*	14	17	12
Male and female friends equally	5	2	2
No one	1	4	6
Number of widowed (= 100%)	347	339	342
Ratio $\dfrac{Female}{Male}$	2.5	2.9	2.1

* Including 'all the family'.

We considered the geographical proximity of relatives and friends, the frequency of contact, and identified the person who was most comfort to the widowed, the person they saw most frequently, and the person who gave them most practical help. *Table 60* shows that daughters were mentioned most often on all three criteria. Female friends were next most likely to be mentioned as the person they saw most often, and sons as the person giving most practical help. The emphasis on females illustrates the expressive role taken on by women, although the relationship found with giving practical help, an instrumental role being traditionally male, is perhaps more unexpected. It is possible, however, that domestic tasks were being referred to by widowed.

On average the widowed mentioned two different people who had helped them in these three different ways. Thirty-four per cent mentioned one person, 37% mentioned two people, 15% three, and 13% four or more. Three people, 1%, identified no one who had helped them in any of these ways.

Those who mentioned just one or two people at these questions had a higher average adjustment score (3.5) than those who mentioned three or more (3.1). There are a number of possible explanations for this difference. One is that more people rallying round and providing support may prevent the widowed spending sufficient time alone to grieve. Another interpretation is that the worse the widowed person's adjustment, the more people rally round and offer support and help. Alternatively, it may simply be that having just one or two people around providing help and support indicates a comparatively close and supportive relationship with the ones they did mention.

Daughters and sons

Given the central role played by daughters and sons in the lives of many of the widowed, it is appropriate to compare those who have daughters and sons with those who do not. Most, 83%, of the widowed had some children; 24% had son(s) only, 21% only daughter(s), and 38% both. *Table 61* suggests that the widowed with daughters only may be more likely to rely on their children for support than those who only had sons. Those without any children were more likely than those with families to turn to siblings, particularly sisters, for help, even though the widowed without children were less likely than those with children to have any siblings who were still alive — 65% in comparison with 79%. And although those with no children were more likely to identify a friend or neighbour rather than a relative as the person they saw most often, they still relied on relatives more often than friends for comfort and practical help.

It was those with no children who were most likely to say no one had comforted them or given them any practical help, and the few who could not identify anyone they saw most often were also childless.

Among those who were disabled in some way,[1] those without any children more often felt they needed help or more help than they were getting: 44% of them felt this compared with 22% of the disabled with children. There was no variation with the sex of children over this.

---

[1] Had difficulty or could not: use public transport, or got out, or go up and down stairs, or get in or out of bath, or dress or undress, or cut toe nails.

Table 61   The supporters of the widowed for those with and without sons and daughters

	Widow or widower has:			
	Son(s) only	Daughter(s) only	Son(s) and daughter(s)	No children
Person most often seen:	%	%	%	%
Son	34	–	17	–
Daughter	–	67	32	–
Brother	1	1	2	11
Sister	7	–	1	11
Other male relative	4	–	1	4
Other female relative	6	3	6	7
Male friend	4	–	4	5
Female friend	27	18	13	43
Other or combinations	17	11	24	14
No one	–	–	–	5
Person most comfort:	%	%	%	%
Son	44	–	11	–
Daughter	–	73	46	–
Brother	2	–	1	4
Sister	7	–	1	14
Other male relative	2	1	2	4
Other female relative	12	7	2	18
Male friend	–	1	1	2
Female friend	13	6	6	31
Other or combinations	14	12	30	11
No one	6	–	–	16
Person most practical help:	%	%	%	%
Son	45	–	20	–
Daughter	–	76	42	–
Brother	4	–	1	2
Sister	6	1	2	13
Other male relative	1	3	2	9
Other female relative	6	5	2	19
Male friend	2	3	1	4
Female friend	19	6	5	21
Other or combinations	13	3	22	11
No one	4	3	3	21
Number of widowed (=100%)	85	73	133	58

Table 62 Frequency of contact with the child, the sibling, and the person they saw most often

	The child:	The sibling:	The person:
	the widowed saw most often		
Frequency of contact:	%	%	%
Daily (including in same household)	31	7	61
More than weekly less than daily	25	10	28
Weekly	12	8	5
More than monthly less than weekly	3	7	2
Monthly	4	6	2
Less than monthly but since death	7	25	1
In year before death	1	4	–
More than a year before death	–	10	–
No children/sibling or person seen most often	17	23	1
Number of widowed (= 100%)	348	343	348

Looking at our adjustment scale there was no significant difference between those with and those without any children, or between those with sons and those with daughters. But more of those with children said they could look forward to things – 37% against 20% of those without any children. It would seem that having children may help adjustment in some ways; 24% of those with children said loneliness was a big problem for them compared with 37% without any children – a difference which did not quite reach the 5% level of significance although, when those with and without any daughters were compared, the difference, 21% against 31%, was more definite. What of the frequency with which they saw their children? This is considered next.

Frequency of contact

Most of the widowed, 68%, saw one of their children at least once a week. Those with children generally saw them with the same frequency as they had done before their spouse died, 53% did so, 36% saw them more often, 8% less frequently, and 3% saw some less often and some more frequently. Contact with siblings was much less frequent but 61% had daily contact with the person they saw most often. The data are in *Table 62*. The widowed were more likely to be in daily contact with a child if they had daughter(s) only (41% in daily contact) than if they had son(s) only (25%). The proportion in daily contact was 43% if they had both son(s) and daughter(s) and this proportion rose with the number of children they had: from 25% of those with one child only, to 38% of those with two or three, to 59% of those with four or more.

The relationship between loneliness and frequency of contact with children is shown in *Table 63*. There is a clear trend in the proportion finding it a big problem, from 17% of those who saw a son or daughter daily to 37% of those who saw one less than weekly. And those who saw one of their children at least once a week had a higher average adjustment score than those who saw their children less frequently (3.5 against 3.0). Those who had children but saw them infrequently — less than once a week — did not differ significantly from the childless in relation to loneliness or adjustment.

The frequency with which they saw their children was not related to the reporting of nerves or depression or their assessment of their health. But the widowed who had less than weekly contact with their children were more likely to say money was a problem for them than

Table 63   Loneliness and most frequent contact with a child

	Frequency of contact with child seen most often:				No children
	Daily	More than weekly, less than daily	Weekly	Less than weekly	
Finds loneliness:	%	%	%	%	%
A big problem	17	20	29	37	37
Intermediate	22	28	29	32	17
No problem	61	52	42	31	46
Number of widowed (= 100%)	107	90	41	51	55

those who had at least weekly contacts, 43% in comparison with 28%. It is possible that they could not afford to make more regular contact, thus feelings of loneliness were enhanced. How much does frequency of contact with other people besides children matter? *Table 64* shows a clear trend: those having daily contact with children had least problem with loneliness and those with no daily contacts with a single person the most, while those with daily contacts with others fell in between.

Table 64   Loneliness and daily contact with children and others

	Child seen every day	Someone other than child seen every day	No one seen every day
Loneliness:	%	%	%
A big problem	17	25	32
Intermediate	22	27	27
No problem	61	48	41
Number of widowed (= 100%)	107	104	133

Berkman and Syme (1979) in a longitudinal study in California found that people who lacked social and community ties were more likely to die in a nine-year follow-up period than those with more extensive contacts; and that contact with close relatives and friends was related to mortality independently of marital status, health, or health habits. Lack of contact is a clear danger signal.

Proximity

As expected the widowed were more likely to see their children if they were living nearby. The relationship is shown in *Table 65*. If their children lived within a half-hour journey almost all the widowed saw them at least once a week, and so did three-fifths of those with children living between half-an-hour and two-hours' journey away. But if the journey was longer than that contact was much less frequent.

As families become smaller and more scattered how many of the widowed have children living near them? Almost two-thirds, 63%,

Table 65 Proximity and frequency of contact with children

| | Nearest child lives: | | | | |
	In same household	Within 10 mins walk	Within ½hr journey	Journey ½hr < 2 hrs	Journey 2 hours+*
Frequency of contact with child seen most often:	%	%	%	%	%
Daily	97	53	14	5	–
Less than daily more than weekly	3	38	52	33	–
Weekly	–	7	26	23	–
More than weekly less than monthly	–	–	4	14	5
Monthly	–	2	3	14	14
Less often	–	–	1	11	81
Number of widowed (=100%)	64	56	102	43	21

* But still in Great Britain.

of the widowed had a child within half-an-hour's journey and two-fifths, 39%, had a sibling as accessible. The importance of accessibility is indicated by the fact that over three-quarters of the people the widowed identified as those who had been most comfort to them and of most practical help since their spouse died lived within half-an-hour's journey. The figures are in *Table 66*. This relationship between proximity of residence and contact with helpers and supporters has been confirmed by Riley and Foner (1968) who found that nearly half of a sample of people aged sixty-five and over drew most of their friends from their own neighbourhood.

Taking the widowed with siblings, those without children were more likely to live within an hour's journey of a sibling than those with children, 80% against 63%, and to have daily contact with siblings, 30% in comparison with 7%. To some extent then, siblings may substitute for children. Cartwright, Hockey, and Anderson (1973) found that ties with brothers and sisters seemed strongest among single people.

What of the wider network of friends, neighbours, and relatives other than children and siblings?

Table 66 The proximity of the child and the sibling the widowed saw most often and the people of most comfort to them and most practical help

	Child sees most often	Sibling sees most often	Person who gave most comfort	Person who gave most practical help
Proximity:	%	%	%	%
Same household	18	2	17	15
Within 10 mins walk	16	13	32	32
Within ½hr journey	29	23	29	29
Journey				
½hr < 1hr	7	15	8	9
1hr < 2hrs	5	8	5	5
2hrs < 4hrs	3	6	4	3
4 hours + but in				
GB	4	7	1	–
Abroad (incl.				
Ireland)	1	3	–	–
No child/sibling/ person who comforts or gives practical help	17	23	4	6
Number of widowed (= 100%)	348	342	338	341

Other relatives, friends, and neighbours

Friends as well as relatives can help by giving support, companion-ship, and understanding. However, Lopata (1973) found that social networks are likely to be disrupted by widowhood. In her study, 38% of widows reported declining social lives while only 12% reported an increase. Friendship interaction was particularly low during the first year of widowhood. We have already shown that contact with children tended to be more frequent rather than less frequent after widowhood. What of their other contacts?

The widowed in the present study were asked if they had seen any other close relatives or good friends besides children and siblings since the death. Seventy-two per cent mentioned someone, and the average number of people mentioned was 1.8. But for over a quarter, children

Table 67   Other close relatives and friends seen since death (besides children and siblings) for those with and those without any children

	Widowed with children	Widowed without living children	All widowed
	%	%	%
Son-in-law	10	2	9
Daughter-in-law	10	–	8
Brother-in-law	11	16	12
Sister-in-law	19	18	19
Grandson	5	–	4
Granddaughter	5	–	4
Other male relative	10	32	14
Other female relative	25	44	28
Male friend	10	18	12
Female friend	23	28	24
No one	29	18	28
Number of widowed (= 100%)	286	57	343

or siblings were the only close relatives they had seen, nor had they seen anyone they regarded as a close friend since their spouse's death. The types of people mentioned are shown in *Table 67*, for those with and those without children. Those without any children more often mentioned other relatives.

Finally, in our attempt to identify the helpers and supporters of the

Table 68   The network of relatives and friends of the widowed

	Proportion of widowed with any	Average number
Children – still alive	83%	1.9
Siblings – still alive	78%	2.1
Other close relatives and good friends seen since death	72%	1.8
Other helpful relatives, friends, or neighbours	42%	0.7
Number of widowed (= 100%)	361	

widowed, we asked if they had any other relatives, friends, or neighbours who had been particularly helpful to them since the death. Over half, 58%, said there was no-one else. Most of those mentioned, 85%, were friends or neighbours rather than relatives. The position is summarized in *Table 68*.

So on average the widowed had a network of 6.5 relatives, friends, and helpers. We have already looked in some detail at the part played by children and siblings, now we consider the role of grandchildren, then neighbours, before going on to examine the association between the different sorts of helpers and supporters, and then any variations between widows and widowers and their age and social class.

Grandchildren

Being a grandparent may be an important source of identity as it is one of the few new roles open to older people. On the other hand, Lopata (1973) found grandparenthood to be of significance in widowhood only if frequent contacts are made between grandchild and grandparent without interference from the child's parents. This, however, rarely happened.

Three-quarters of the widowed in the present study had grandchildren. Almost a quarter, 24%, had one or two, 21% had three or four, and 29% had five or more. Most of the widowed, 80%, had seen all their grandchildren since the death and 18% had seen some. Two per cent had not seen any. So most of the widowed were in contact with their grandchildren, although as we saw earlier few mentioned them spontaneously as close relatives to whom they looked for help and support. But some commented that having grandchildren helped or comforted them:

'They've [daughter and husband] had two babies this year. It's helped a great deal having them to think about.'

Others mentioned babysitting for their sons and daughters:

'I do have the kiddies sometimes while my daughter goes to town.'

One widow was highly involved with her grandchildren now as her daughter-in-law had died in the previous year, leaving three children, aged 7, 11, and 15. This widow travelled thirty miles four days a week to help her son look after them. But she enjoyed doing this and it helped occupy her:

'I help with the grandchildren from Tuesday to Friday each week. I'm always trying to help, wherever and whenever I can. I like to do it.'

No relationship was found between contact with grandchildren and loneliness or adjustment to widowhood.

Neighbours

Neighbours may be able to provide the widowed with a sense of security as well as being a source of immediate help and support. Lopata (1973) found that widows turn to their neighbours when they become lonely as a result of bereavement, while later either other relations may take over, or the widow withdraws into isolation. We asked the widowed how well they knew their neighbours. Over half, 59%, said they knew them 'very well', 20% 'fairly well', 17% 'just a little', while 4% did not know them at all. The widowed often indicated that their neighbours gave them companionship or comfort:

'She [neighbour] used to look in when my wife was alive. I go and sit with her now. We're both lonely, she's a widow. We sit and look out of the window at the view.'

'I don't know what I would have done without them. Nancy knows where the key is. She watches to see if my curtains are drawn back before she goes to work. . . . My husband used to look after me if I had a heart attack. He would take care of me until I felt better. I soon recover. Nancy would come in to me if I was taken bad again.'

'Molly next door. She's been here about as long as I have. She calls over the 'phone every day to see if I'm allright. She's eighty − a widow like me.'

'I see my widowed neighbour every day. We keep a check on each other to make sure we're all right, she's been widowed twelve years, and there's Henry next door. He said "Knock on the wall if you need some help". It's very nice to know you've got someone close by if you need help.'

Those who lived in houses or bungalows were more likely than those in flats or rooms to say they knew their neighbours 'very well': 62% in comparison with 42%.

It is possible that neighbourliness, amongst other things, can help people adjust better to the death of their spouse, perhaps by lessening feelings of isolation or aloneness. There was some suggestion that those who knew their neighbours either 'very well' or 'fairly well' were less likely to find loneliness a big problem − 23% of them did so compared with 35% of those who knew their neighbours less well or not at all. But this difference might have arisen by chance. There was however a significant difference with our adjustment scale: those who knew their neighbours 'very well' had an average score of 3.5 compared with 3.2 for those who knew them less well or not at all, while those who had been given some help by their neighbours scored 3.6 on average against 3.3 for those who had not had any help. In addition, more of the widowed who knew their neighbours well expected to stay in their present home for the rest of their lives: the proportion who thought they would do so fell from 63% of those who knew their neighbours 'very well' to 50% of those who knew them 'just a little' or not at all. Among all the widowed over half, 54%, said they would miss their neighbours 'a lot' if they moved away, 19% said they would miss them 'a little', and 26% said they would not miss them at all.

Apart from companionship it was practical help that neighbours often provided. Two-thirds of the widowed said they had had some help from neighbours either before or since their spouse died.[2] To what extent did neighbours and other relatives and friends act as alternative sources of support for those without children or siblings?

Network associations

Earlier in this chapter we looked at the widowed with, and those without, any children and saw that although the childless were less likely to have any siblings, as a group they saw more of their brothers and sisters and relied on them more for both comfort and practical help. Friends were also more important in these respects for the childless than for those with children (see *Table 61*).

No differences were found between those who had children and those who did not with how well they knew their neighbours. Nor were the widowed living alone any more likely to know their neighbours well. On the other hand those without children were more likely to have had some help from neighbours − 83% of them had received some help either before or since their spouse's death compared with 60% of those with children. This suggests that the childless have to

[2] 'Did any of them (neighbours) help you at all, either before —— died or since then?'

rely for help on people they know less well. So although siblings may substitute for children to some extent and both friends and neighbours for relatives, the support network of the childless is less well defined. Whereas 16% of the childless could not identify any one person whom they saw at least once a week, only 4% of those with children were in that situation. More of the childless as we will show later were isolated.

But the childless identified more close relatives (other than children or siblings) and good friends with whom they had been in contact since their spouse died, than did the widowed with children: the average numbers were 2.5 and 1.8 respectively. A similar difference existed in the numbers of other helpers they identified: for these the averages were 1.0 for the childless compared with 0.7 for those with children. A comparison of those with and without siblings showed no such differences, but as we showed earlier contact with siblings was much less frequent than with children.

Variations with sex, age, and social class

Sex

Widows and widowers did not differ significantly in the proportion living with children, nor in the distance between them and their nearest child. They also saw one of their children as frequently. In addition, both widows and widowers relied more on daughters than sons for comfort and practical help and they saw daughters more frequently than sons.

Over siblings the situation was rather different. Although the widowers in our sample were rather older on average than the widows they did not differ in the number of siblings that were still alive. But widows saw a sibling more often than widowers: 19% of the former saw a brother or sister more than once a week, 12% of the latter. This could not be explained by any difference in the proximity of siblings.

Widows also seemed to have closer ties with neighbours than widowers. Sixty-two per cent of widows said they knew their neighbours 'very well' compared with 51% of widowers, and 68% of widows, 57% of widowers had had some help from neighbours, although this last difference might have occurred by chance. They did not differ in the numbers of other close relatives, good friends or, other helpers which they identified but the sex ratio of the other close relatives and good friends they had seen since their spouse's death was different. Widows had seen 2.6 females to every one male, widowers 1.3.

So we have found some differences between widows and widowers in their contacts with siblings and neighbours, but no clear differences between them in the indicators we found were related to loneliness: that is, frequency of contact with children and daily contact with a single person. And we saw earlier that there were no significant differences in the proportions finding loneliness a big problem, or a problem at all.

Age

Increasing age, as well as increasing frailty, and declining health, was not associated with more frequent contact with children. Those aged seventy-five or over were less likely to have any siblings still alive: 68% of them compared with 82% of the younger widowed. They were also less likely to have seen other close relatives (besides children or siblings) or good friends since their spouse's death: 63% of these older widowed had done so, 77% of the others. So children did not compensate for a declining circle of close relatives and friends or declining mobility by seeing elderly widowed parents more often than younger ones. Nevertheless those aged seventy-five or more were as likely as younger ones to see someone every day, although they were no more or less likely to have had help from neighbours.

Social class

The working-class widowed had larger families than middle-class ones – that is they had both more children and more siblings. They were also more likely to see a child daily, a sibling at least weekly, and to live nearer to them. The details are in *Table 69*. To what extent is their greater proximity and frequency of contact simply a reflection of their larger family size? It can be seen from the table that it is not just a function of having children or siblings.

Further analyses are difficult because of the small numbers involved, but they suggest that class differences in proximity to children may be largely explained by the differences in the numbers of children, while within each family size the working-class widowed

Table 69   Social class and family size, proximity, and frequency of contact with children and siblings

	Middle-class widowed	Working-class widowed
All widowed:		
Average number of children	1.5	2.2
Proportion with child within ½-hr journey	52%	68%
Proportion seeing a child daily	18%	36%
Proportion with any children	80%	85%
Widowed with children only:		
Average number of children	1.9	2.6
Proportion with a child within ½-hr journey	65%	81%
Proportion seeing a child daily	23%	42%
All widowed:		
Average number of siblings	1.7	2.2
Proportion with a sibling within ½-hr journey	27%	42%
Proportion seeing a sibling at least weekly	14%	29%
Proportion with any sibling	70%	81%
Widowed with any siblings:		
Average number of siblings	2.4	2.7
Proportion with a sibling within ½-hr journey	38%	53%
Proportion seeing a sibling at least weekly	20%	36%
Number of widowed	95	263
Number of widowed with child(ren)	74	214
Number of widowed with sibling(s)	64	202

may be rather more likely to see a child daily. The figures relating to this last assertion are in *Table 70* — but though consistent do not reach a level of statistical significance. However, the observed differences gain in credence by a comparison of the working- and middle-class widowed whose nearest child lived between ten minutes and half an hour's journey away. None of the middle class in this

184   Life After A Death

Table 70   Daily contact with children by class and family size

	Proportion seeing a child each day	
	Middle class	Working class
Number of children:		
One	18% (34)	29% (63)
Two	21% (19)	43% (68)
Three or four	32% (19)	41% (58)

Figures in brackets are numbers on which percentages are based (= 100%).

situation saw a child daily, compared with 18% of the working class.

With siblings it was only possible (because of the numbers involved) to compare those with just one sibling still alive, and here a significant difference emerged: the working-class widowed were more likely to live within half-an-hour's journey of their surviving sibling than middle-class ones – 55% compared with 26%. This picture of kinship solidarity, or lack of mobility, among the working classes has also been found by Townsend (1957) and Willmott and Young (1960).

The middle class seemed to compensate to some extent for their smaller families and less frequent contact with children and siblings by their friendship network. They more often mentioned a friend as the person they saw most frequently: 41% compared with 26% of the working-class widowed said this, and the middle class more frequently got most practical help from a friend, 21% against 12% of the working class. In addition, more of the middle-class than working-class widowed identified friends they had found particularly helpful: 48% compared with 34%. But although the middle class had a wider network of friends they did not seem to have closer relationships with neighbours: they did not know them better nor were they any more likely to have any help from them. Finally, with these different network patterns there were no class differences in the proportion in daily contact with a single person nor in the proportion finding loneliness a problem.

Isolation

Up to now we have been looking at the contact between the elderly widowed and their relatives and friends and the comfort and help this

gives them. But what of those who are isolated, who have few contacts? In this section we consider various groups who might be thought
of as isolated in different ways, starting with those who live alone.

Living alone

In Chapter 4, we saw that most of the widowed, 78%, were living
alone, and nowadays living alone is a frequent experience for the
elderly. So those who are isolated in this sense are by no means a
deviant group, although, as we showed earlier, many of them found
living alone difficult to accept, and problems of loneliness were more
common among this group though not confined to them.

What contacts did those living alone have with other people? Half
of them were in daily contact with the person they saw most often,
while a further 36% saw someone more than weekly, 6% someone
weekly, but 8% did not see any one person even as often as once a
week. In spite of this relative lack of contact — since nearly all those
living in a household saw someone every day — those living alone had
a similar score on our adjustment scale to those living with others. But
what is the effect of having relatively infrequent contact with people?

Infrequent contact

Altogether thirty-seven widows and widowers, 11%, could be defined
as relatively isolated in that they did not see any one person more than
once a week. Two comments about this were:

> 'The people who live round here don't come and see me. Nobody's
> come and spoken to me today and I don't suppose I shall talk to
> anyone for the rest of the day.'

> 'You could die and nobody would know.'

Who were these isolated widowed? No differences were found with
background factors such as sex, social class, age, or health; nor did
they differ in their number of siblings. However 27% of the isolated
group compared with 15% of the other widowed had no living
children — a suggestive difference which did not quite reach the level
of statistical significance. The isolated had a relatively low adjustment score: 2.9 on average compared with 3.4 for the others. But they
were no more likely to report problems with nerves or depression,

although 64% of them compared with 45% of the others said lone-liness was a problem for them. There were a few, 4% of the widowed, who did not see anyone more often than once a month. Three of these seemed particularly isolated, although they all had a child who lived within half-an-hour's journey. One woman had six children and one sister but only saw them either monthly or less often, even though one son and daughter lived within ten minutes' walk. She said she saw them infrequently because they worked. Apart from her doctor her only other visitor was the health visitor who had been to see her about getting a home help. She lived in a block of old people's flats and found it 'too quiet'. She refused to sit in the communal lounge pro-vided as she said: 'I don't want to sit with elderly people.' She con-tinued:

> 'It's a funny thing with these flats, none of them seem to have visitors. Some of them sit in there [communal lounge] to save their electricity. I like the flat but not the environment.'

She said living alone was 'terrible' and she found it very difficult to accept. She had lived there for between two and five years and regretted leaving her old neighbours:

> 'In my old home the neighbours brought in things and gave me messages and I did the same. You can't pick and choose neigh-bours. I made a mistake.'

One of her daughters had suggested the widow move in with her but the widow found the grandchildren 'too boisterous'. Her main problem, she said, was 'lack of friends'. She said she had 'nothing to look forward to', did not think she would come to terms with the death, and felt things were 'not going at all well'. One problem was her difficulty going out:

> 'I'm frightened to go out in case my knees give way, but you never get anywhere by staying in.'

Another widow had two daughters and two siblings and her most frequent contact with anyone was with her daughters whom she saw monthly. One lived between half-an-hour and an hour's journey away and the other lived between one and two hour's journey away. She said she did not see the nearest daughter very often as she did not get on with her son-in-law. She said she felt he treated her like dirt. She was lonely, did not look forward to things in the same way, had not come to terms with the death, and felt things were not going very well. Her main problem, she said, was difficulty meeting people:

'I'd like to join in more clubs but how does one meet people when it all costs so much money? How do people get to know you need help? Other people seem to get help round here but no one calls on me.'

However, she was in contact with her doctor and had been visited by a social worker. She said she did not want any other official visitors – just friends.

The third, also a widow, had one sister, an ex-sister-in-law, and one son. Her most frequent contact was with the son whom she saw monthly, although he lived within half-an-hour's journey away. She said he had 'dropped out':

'He moves from lodging-house to lodging-house. I never know how to find him.'

Of her sister and sister-in-law she said:

'My sister is in the home for the blind. She's a bit simple too, always has been. She's been in the school since she was sixteen. I can't bother Sheila [ex-sister-in-law]. . . . She has a new life to make with her new husband.'

This widow, too, found loneliness a problem, did not look forward to things, had not come to terms with the death, and wanted to change some parts of her life – 'to get my son settled again'. She had never consulted her doctor and her only official visitor was the insurance man.

Others led isolated lives apparently largely by choice:

'I've never been asked out anywhere. Only once in my life have I been asked out and that was to tea with some friends – only once in forty-seven years.'

This widow might be described as a loner:

'In a way I've always lived alone. I'm myself. I'm quite happy with my own company. I keep myself busy. . . . I'm quite capable of looking after myself. . . . I haven't seen a doctor for thirty years.'

She had no children, siblings, close relatives, or good friends, and did not identify anyone who had comforted her or given her any practical help. But when asked about her neighbours she said she knew:

'Just the lady opposite. She's seventy-seven years old. She does the odd bit of shopping for me. But not my next door neighbours, they move so frequently. Now I know Mr and Mrs ——. They live quite near. . . . I got asked (out for a meal) once but I didn't go. It was my neighbour who asked me to lunch, but I didn't want to go.'

Others, by contrast, had more frequent contacts with people but felt neglected.

The neglected

We asked the widowed if there was any one relative or friend they would particularly like to see, or to see more often. Twenty-nine per cent said there was. Sons were mentioned by 7%, daughters by 4%, siblings by 11%, other relatives by 8%, and friends by 4%. Those who felt neglected in this way had a relatively low adjustment score: an average of 3.1 compared with 3.5 for the others; felt more lonely – 59% of them against 42% of the others said this was a problem; and more of them reported problems with nerves or depression – 60% against 41% – and sleeplessness – 59% against 47%.

Keeping in touch with friends and relatives may involve financial outlays if travel costs are involved. And there may be other problems in travelling:

'I'd like to see all my friends more often really and my cousin-in-law. It takes time and petrol to get there, she lives in ——. She needs to see me too, life's not very easy for her.'

Ill health and increasing age also presented difficulties:

'A lot of my sisters (I am one of nine) are too ill to come and visit me now.'

'Her [wife's] three brothers. They're getting older now. They can't get out and nor can I.'

But some just felt neglected. One widow would have liked to have seen her husband's brothers but said 'They don't want to'. She went on:

'I dread to ask my relatives. I asked if I could go to Wales to stay with one of my brothers-in-law. At first they said "Yes" and I started packing my things. Then they rang my cousin to say they couldn't take me. I rang his sister to ask if I could go there for a few days but she said "No".'

In a number of ways this widow seemed quite embittered:

'People don't want you around these days. . . . Sometimes I wish I wouldn't wake up in the morning.'

When the interviewer was leaving she told her that the doctor at the hospital had asked her if she had ever thought of taking her own life:

'I just looked at him and said no, I have not. He was trying to catch me. If I'd said yes he might have had me taken away.'

She had no children but a brother and a cousin both of whom she saw more than once a week.

Another widow would have liked to see more of her only son and of her one brother but 'they are so far away and travelling is so expensive'. She went on to say:

'Nobody can help me. Who can help me? You think you are alone, you feel terrible. You are so alone, so lost.'

She had been visited by a vicar but felt he was of little help:

'People haven't got the time. He [vicar] wanted to be out before he was in − busy, busy, busy.'

Finally one widower who had not identified anyone who had comforted him or given him any practical help and who said the person he saw most often was his sister whom he saw less than monthly, also said there were no other relatives or friends he would particularly like to see, but in describing how he felt about living alone he said:

'I don't care much about it. I've always been used to a lot of company. I've been a mixer.'

And later in the interview:

'I still feel lost. I've no one to turn to.'

Summary

Most widows and widowers obtained emotional, social, and practical support from their network of relatives and friends. This chapter has shown the important part played by children, particularly daughters, in providing this support. Even though just a small proportion of older widowed people live with their children, many more live relatively near them and interact frequently. Proximity was important, but most of those who did not have children living near got support from other relatives or friends. Frequent contact with someone close to them appeared to relieve some of the feelings of loneliness.

But some of the widowed did not have a supportive network. We looked at three indicators of possible isolation: living alone, not being in contact with any one person at least once a week, and feeling neglected. The first, and most common one, living alone, was not related to our measure of adjustment, but the neglected and those infrequently in contact with others appeared to be less well adjusted to their widowhood. A few seemed isolated by choice, others by circumstances. In the final chapter we will be looking at what can be done to identify and help the neglected and at how the numbers of those isolated by circumstances might be reduced. But before that we consider the viewpoint of their supporters.

9 The impact on the familiars

In the last chapter we saw how elderly widowed people depended on their relatives and friends, and that these relationships were important in helping them to adjust to their new situation and to overcome their feelings of loneliness and isolation. What does this mean to the people they turn to for support and help? In this chapter we look at the experiences and views of the widowed people's familiars — those they identified as knowing most about their circumstances since their bereavement.

Who were these people? Earlier we showed that most, 69%, were women, almost half, 46%, being daughters. Daughters outnumbered sons by two to one. One in eight of the familiars were elderly, aged sixty-five or more, themselves. Most, four-fifths, were married and nearly two-fifths had young children, under fifteen. So a sizeable minority had the dual role of looking after their young families and providing support for the widowed, and earlier many of them had been involved in caring for the spouse who died. One familiar described the conflicting commitments:

> 'I have young children and I couldn't stretch myself enough. I had to give constant care to my mother and put her first which was difficult. The family grumbled and got very upset.'

A number of familiars had a further commitment — employment. Almost half worked full-time and a quarter worked part-time. Eighty-six per cent of the men worked full-time in comparison with 26% of the women.

192   Life After A Death

Contact with the widowed and practical help

Fourteen per cent of the familiars lived in the same household as the widow or widower, a further 22% were in daily contact with them, and another 52% saw them weekly or more often, leaving 12% who saw them less often or irregularly. If telephone contacts are included the proportion either living with or in daily contact with the widowed rises to 46% with a further 50% in at least weekly contact. But of course 40% of the widowed did not have a telephone; if they wanted to talk to relatives or friends on the phone they had to depend on neighbours with a 'phone or use a public one. A few familiars described how they found the widowed person's dependence an embarrassment. One, a friend, had avoided giving the widow his home telephone number as she demanded so much attention:

> 'She wants my 'phone number at home but I won't give it to her. She's always ringing here [work] to ask for it. . . . She talks an awful lot so the person on the other end just does all the listening and has to be passive.'

Two-fifths of the familiars lived either with the widow or widower or within walking distance of their home, but some, 16%, had journeys of half an hour or more, and for 28% the cost was 50p or more each time they met. (For further details see Bowling, in draft.)

Apart from being in touch with the widowed person what other help and support did the familiars give? To some extent this depended on the level of physical dependency of the widowed and their need for emotional support. Most of the familiars, 63%, helped the widowed with household tasks,[1] particularly shopping, 32%; washing clothes, 27%; odd jobs, 29%; cooking and preparing food, 18%; and gardening, 17%. Although the familiars felt they were the most common source of help with these tasks, they reported that other relatives helped 55% of the widowed and other friends or neighbours 28%. Nearly half, 45%, were said to have a home or paid help – usually with cleaning windows – while 8% were said to have no help at all with these tasks. But 24% of the widowed were felt by the familiars to need help with household tasks that they were not getting – mainly with cleaning their homes and with gardening. The familiars themselves

[1] Shopping, preparing/cooking food, washing up, making beds, cleaning house, washing clothes, cleaning windows, gardening, odd jobs around the house.

were giving some help to two-thirds of these widows and widowers, but did not feel they could help enough or in ways that were needed. So there was some anxiety about the widowed person's ability to cope with practical tasks. These are illustrated by two comments:

> 'He wouldn't accept help but he really needed it. The house was a tip. I (daughter) was trying to get him a flat when he died (nine months after his wife).'

> 'He's not managing well with his life at all. He won't cook for himself and if he does he won't eat it.'

We also asked familiars about the ways in which they helped the widowed with more personal tasks and with getting around.[2] Forty-three per cent of the widowed were thought by the familiars to have problems with some of these other tasks or to need help with them. (This is similar to the proportion of widowed who themselves said they had this sort of problem, 41%). Again the familiars felt themselves to be the most usual source of support, and 15% of them helped the widowed in these ways. One in ten felt the widowed could do with more of this sort of help. This may also have been a source of anxiety.

Further indication of the dependence of the disabled widowed on relatives and friends comes from an analysis of their sources of help. These were categorized into relatives, friends or neighbours, and others. Of the seventy-seven sources mentioned as helping with using public transport, going out, going up and down stairs, getting in or out of bath, dressing and undressing, 61% were relatives, 27% friends or neighbours, and 12% others – mainly paid professional help. For cutting toe nails the situation was quite different, the most common source of help mentioned here, by 71% of those receiving any, was a chiropodist but 23% had help with this from a relative.

Restrictions on the lives of the familiars

What effect did the help and support the familiars gave to the widowed have on their own lives? In reply to an open question about how the help and support they had given the widowed had affected their lives the following types of responses were given:

> 'I haven't been out anywhere for maybe fourteen months, maybe

[2] Using public transport, going out, going up and down stairs, getting in and out of bath, dressing and undressing, cutting toe nails.

longer. . . . Sometimes I feel so low I cry every night. Mum doesn't know that though. We have to use my money because Mum's only got one pension now.'

'I feel a lot less relaxed now than I did before we lived together [moved in with widow after the death]. I seem to be on edge a bit more which isn't me. . . . I don't feel as free obviously. It's a little bit like being married. You've someone else to consider.'

'Whereas you'd sit down at night I've gone up to mother to sit with her. You don't find time to do things you'd want to do.'

'It makes for problems. My husband gets angry. He says I've given far too much time to my parents. I can't get to see elderly in-laws and other friends as much as I'd like. I pay for a lot of extra things for him [widower], especially food, and I also pay for his laundry. It's aged me and taken away a lot of the joy of living.'

'Just being responsible for her really and having to be with her. I was just getting independent myself with the boys growing up. Now that's gone.'

On the other hand, some familiars said they were closer to the widowed now because of the help and support they had given him or her:

'It's just made me closer to her. We had tended to drift apart because of distance and so on, but this happening has renewed the friendship.'

'I think we're closer now. I didn't get on too well with my Dad before.'

We asked them whether they had given up or cut down on any of their social activities – such as visiting friends or relatives (12% had given up or cut down on this), going out to other social activities (13%), going on holiday (7%), and entertaining people at home (9%). Altogether 7% had given up at least one of these things and a further 14% had cut down on them.

We also asked about the effects the help and support they had given the widowed had had on other, more personal, aspects of their lives. Ten per cent of familiars said it had affected their relationships with relatives, friends, or neighbours; 18% mentioned their health; 9% their income; and 12% said it had affected the amount of help they were able to give other people. Seventy per cent said it had not

Table 71   Some factors related to the impact on the familiar

	Proportion of familiars:			Number of familiars (=100%)
	Who had given up or cut down on doing certain things	Who felt life had been affected	Whose activities had been restricted	
Familiar reported that:				
Mobility of widowed caused				
Some difficulty	29%	39%	38%	92
No problem	14%	24%	23%	119
Widowed had difficulty with personal tasks				
Yes	33%	43%	42%	83
No	14%	24%	23%	119
Loneliness a problem for widowed				
Yes	22% ⎫*	31%	38%	134
No	19% ⎭	19%	16%	75
Widowed depressed				
Yes	26%	41%	41%	121
No	13%	15%	14%	87
Widowed had come to terms with death				
No	27% ⎫*	38%	41%	44
Yes	19% ⎭	27%	26%	158
Widowed person's age:				
Under 65	16% ⎫*	19%	24% ⎫*	37
65 or more	22% ⎭	33%	30% ⎭	174
Sex of familiar:				
Male	12%	15%	18%	66
Female	25%	37%	34%	145
Relationship of familiar to widowed:				
Son or daughter	24% ⎫*	36%	35%	147
Other	15% ⎭	17%	16%	64
Familiar lives with widowed:				
Yes	40%	43% ⎫*	50%	30
No	18%	28% ⎭	26%	181

* Not significant at the 5% level.

affected any of these things. Finally, we asked about restrictions on their activities. Fourteen per cent said their activities had been severely or fairly restricted, 15% a little restricted, and 71% said they had not been at all restricted.

Table 71 shows that the impact on the familiars was greater when, according to familiars, the widowed had problems with mobility[3] and personal tasks[4] and when the familiar felt there were problems with emotional adjustment. The table also shows that women and children of the widowed suffered more restrictions than other familiars, as did those who lived with the widowed. Further analyses showed clearly that a heavy burden fell on the familiars who were daughters. It was found that daughters of the widowed were more likely to have given up something because of the care and support they gave the widowed than other familiars, 28% in comparison with 15%. Daughters of the widowed were also more likely than others to say their lives had been affected, 46% against 17%, and to say that their lives had been restricted, 44% compared with 17%.

The number of familiars who were 'burdened' according to at least one of the three measures used — given up or cut down on something, affects on life, and life restrictions — was 86, or 41%. This total group of 'burdened' familiars were more likely to be women, 79% in comparison with 61% of other familiars, and they were more likely to be daughters of the widowed, 65% in comparison with 31%. In addition they were probably more likely to live with the widowed, 20% in comparison with 10% of other familiars, although this last difference might have arisen by chance. In the next section we look at the experience of those who lived in the same home as the widowed in more detail.

The home sharers

Two-thirds of the thirty familiars who lived with the widowed were daughters; half these daughters had never married and had lived with their parents for all their lives, most of the others were married (one was divorced) and had only started to live with their mother or father again since the death of their other parent. In contrast all the seven sons who lived with the widowed were single and had been living at home for all their lives, or in one instance for at least twenty years.

---

[3] Using public transport, going out, going up and down stairs, getting in and out of bath.

[4] Dressing and undressing, cutting toe nails.

Just over two-fifths of these familiars lived only with the widow or widower. These were mostly single children. One in ten lived with their spouse and the widow or widower, a fifth shared their home with the widowed person, their spouse, and their children.

Responses to an open question about how they felt about sharing a home with the widowed varied from 'happy' and 'I have always done it so it is no different' to:

'I'm finding it very difficult of course. Not having any children, having a third person here makes a big difference. We've never had anyone else living with us and you really notice a third person always there.'

'I'm bitter because although he's in good health he expects to be waited on hand and foot.'

'Sometimes you get a bit fed up and things start boiling up.'

Just over three-quarters of this small group said, in reply to a direct question, that the widowed got on with them and their families 'very well' and just under a fifth said 'fairly well'. Only one, a daughter, said they did not get on very well. She felt 'bitter', and said this was because her father 'wants it all his own way':

'He's on to a good thing. He has a room to himself, he's well fed. He's nothing to complain about.'

The widower himself similarly said that he had 'everything', although his view was that there were no problems in sharing a home and that he got on with his daughter and her family 'very well'.

We asked familiars whether there was anything they or their families could not do or had to because of sharing a home with the widowed person. Just under one in five said there were things they could not do and slightly less than one in ten said there were things they had to do that they would rather not do because of sharing a home. Some comments were:

'I feel I'm a prisoner in my own home. I can't tell him what to do because he is my father.'

'We can't just get up and go out together. We have to go out separately or make arrangements.'

'It's difficult for us to go out and leave her alone for instance.

I like to play golf but I can't go and leave her for five hours at a time. She's very nervous being alone.'

'My husband agreed to give up his [twin] bed so she could be with me in the same room.'

'He is a responsibility. I have merely stepped into my mother's shoes. It can be very difficult. The demands are very great.'

'A fortnight after they came I'd been after a job I wanted — then I couldn't take it.'

'We have disagreements every now and then but no stand-up rows. Financially I'm paying out more than before. Whatever I buy for the house I never ask my mum to contribute to it. I think every now and then you wish you were on your own in your own house, mainly because of my little girl — sometimes my mum wants to interfere.'

We asked the ten who had shared a home with the widowed person during the last year only, whether they came to live with the widowed or whether the widowed came to live with them. For nine the move was made by the widowed or couple and in one case both the familiar and the widow had moved. Most of the moves were local: three were less than a mile and another three were less than 5 miles. One move was between 20 and 60 miles away from the previous home and three moves were further than this.

What were the reasons for the move? Familiars said the widowed person was either too ill to live alone, could not cope with living alone, or could not face it:

'I wanted her here to look after her because she was so ill.'

'She just couldn't live alone. She couldn't really cope even when my father was ill.'

'She couldn't face going back home after he died. She just couldn't imagine being on her own. She was so upset at first. She was continually crying. I thought she was going to have a nervous breakdown. But being with us she made an effort not to make us upset. I could hear her crying in bed at night though when she felt no one was listening.'

One woman, the widow's niece, let the widow stay with her as there was nowhere else for her to go:

'Because her daughter wouldn't have her any longer. She couldn't cope with illness. I felt that there was no choice. I couldn't let her go into a home.'

When asked if their lives had changed at all or been affected by the move or change, nine of the ten familiars said 'Yes'. Eight of these were children of the widowed. However, seven were glad about the move or change while three had mixed feelings about it.[5] One familiar said things were better now:

'It's changed for the better. Now I've a constant babysitter. I can go out with my husband any time, and now I can go out to work too. She helps with the housework and when I get home from work everything is done and the meal is ready. Everything is much easier for me now.'

Another said the burden on her had eased because of the move:

'It's difficult to say because my husband retired at the same time. It's quite different really. I'm quite pleased really. It's relieved me because I don't have to worry about two houses to look after. She's under my eye. I don't have to worry if she's all right.'

For four others, however, the restrictions were greater now, although they all said they were glad about the move or change.

Future problems

As care of the elderly is often a long-term commitment, we asked respondents if they saw any, or any other, problems for themselves, or their families, because of the help or support the widowed might need in the future. Thirty-seven per cent said 'Yes'. Problems arising from the worsening health of the widowed or the possibility of the widowed moving in with the familiar were among the things mentioned:

'If she comes to live here then I have a problem because I shall have to pack up my job and be confined to the house 24 hours a day.'

'When he goes downhill, and he's had one stroke, it (the caring process) could start all over again.'

'If she became ill it would be a problem. I couldn't afford to give up working until the boys left school.'

[5] 'So on balance are you: Glad about the move/change, sorry about the move/change, or do you have mixed feelings about it?'

'There are going to be problems. One day he is not going to be able to be on his own and will have to live with someone – us or my brother-in-law.'

Familiars were asked whether they or the widowed had talked at all about the possibility of the widowed moving from his or her present home. Most of the familiars who had discussed such a possibility (three-fifths) were in favour of the move. One such, a brother of the widower who wanted to move in with him, said:

'I'm sixty-five and my brother [widower] is in a state [of poor health]. I couldn't cope with looking after the farm, and running the house, and seeing to my brother.'

Other comments made by familiars were:

'He'd be much nearer if he wanted us [if he moved]. We could keep an eye on him. He could babysit.'

'It's a long story. I always promised my mother that I would move down to —— when the girls left home. My youngest daughter was married this year and with father dying my mother expected me to move down. But there aren't any jobs in that area and I must work. I've asked my mother to move back up here but she won't. It reminds her of poverty and hard times. Down there she has a dif-ferent sort of life – all her friends from the WI and the church are there.'

'I probably wouldn't be able to put friends up then [if the widower moved in]. I go out to work too so I might feel guilty about that, especially if he was ill.'

The feelings of the familiars

Familiars were asked how they felt about the amount of help they had given to the widowed: 'When someone is widowed, people or other relatives sometimes expect relatives or friends to do too much for the widow (or widower). Have you felt that anyone expected you to do too much in any way?' Thirteen per cent said 'Yes' to this. We asked them who expected it and why they thought they were expected to do too much. The types of replies given are illustrated by the following state-ments. Although no statistically significant differences were found with this and the marital status or relationship to the widowed, some familiars did blame these characteristics − being the un-married daughter, or simply the only daughter − for their burden:

'The sheer fact of Mum's nature, and the fact that I was un-attached, made me the obvious target.'

'People think I'm capable of taking on anything and leave me to do it. I feel I'm a nervous wreck. It's made me very bitter. It all falls on me being the only female.'

Some familiars felt the widow or widower expected too much from them:

'She's so demanding, always wanting me round there so that she can talk all the time about herself. It's very selfish.'

'I think Mum expects too much sometimes. She relies on me too much. She cries a lot, we both do. She expects a lot of help. When I come home at night I don't have much rest.'

Others simply blamed the 'uncaring' or 'selfish' attitudes of other relatives:

'We have always done it and this has just increased since Dad died. They [brothers] are too self-centred − too busy running their own lives. Dad used to sit and cry because the lads never went down to see him when he was ill.'

'Her sisters and her brother − I think they should have 'phoned her more often and written to her. None of them rang her or got in touch except to come to the funeral. None of them have lost a spouse and until they do I don't think you realize how much the bereaved person needs support and contact.'

'Her two sons. I think they could have gone more. They've been down twice in seventeen years. I wonder if it's their wives. It may be lack of thought. I've had a row with them and I told them they were selfish.'

Women were more likely than men to feel that there was someone who should have helped more, 32% in comparison with 20%. And those who thought too much was expected of them were more likely to feel their lives had been affected by looking after the widowed, 61% of them felt this compared with 25% of other familiars, and to say their activities had been restricted, 46% against 26%.

What about mental strains? We asked familiars if they ever worried

or felt anxious about the widowed. Two-thirds said they did. Loneliness, the possibility of something happening to the widowed when he
or she was alone, poor health, and immobility were among the things
mentioned:

> 'Most of the time — because she's on her own and not very happy.
> And at her age she can do silly things.'
>
> 'Sometimes I sit down and I think "God, he's up there, you know,
> all on his own".'
>
> 'All the time I'm out of the house. It's because she's so nervous.'

Another familiar said the worry and support was making her feel
irritable and upset:

> 'It has made me very irritable and tearful and I get a bit nasty and
> bad tempered with the family. I take it out on them. My husband
> realizes why it is. I am feeling sorry for myself. I cry my eyes out.'

In reply to a direct question, over a quarter, 28%, of familiars
mentioned relatives, friends, or neighbours who they felt should have
helped or helped more. Among the reasons given for their not helping
were that people had lost touch over the years, they were too busy
working or looking after their families, or that they were too selfish or
uncaring:

> 'Since Dad died they [widow's two sons] have never asked her to
> their house and have never had her to dinner. One of my brothers
> had a fortnight's holiday at home and never once asked her to go
> out with them for a ride. And my other brother always has an
> excuse that he is doing something in the house. He says he won't
> fetch her and she has got to come up and see him on the bus. I
> tackled him because this has brought problems to the family since
> Dad died. Mum comes crying to me and so I had to ask them about
> it. He told me that unfortunately I was the eldest daughter and it
> was going to fall to me as he and his wife like to be on their own! I
> blew my top!'

And earlier, in Chapter 5, we saw that one in eight of the familiars felt
the widow or widower was not getting the support they needed from
their general practitioner.

So although the majority of the familiars were quite prepared to support and help the widowed, there was a certain amount of resentment

about the amount of support they were expected to give and the failure, as they saw it, of both informal networks and formal services to provide adequate care.

One problem, as we explained in our introduction, is that we may not have seen some of the familiars who gave most help as the widowed seemed anxious to protect them from further tasks such as answering our questions. There is the additional problem that a few widows and widowers, 4% of our initial sample, were said by the people our interviewers contacted to be too ill, confused, or upset to take part in our study. The people looking after them gave us some limited information about the widowed person's situation. This is described next as these elderly widowed people were clearly in need of substantial help.

The care of the widowed who were too unfit to take part in our study

The numbers of these were small, but their 'case histories' give some indication of the problems encountered by the people who were looking after them. Six of the nineteen were in a hospital or other institution – four in an old people's home, one in a psychiatric hospital, and one in a psychiatric ward of a general hospital. All six had been in such institutions before the death of their spouse. The other thirteen either lived in their own homes (6), or in the home of the supporter interviewed (4), or of another relative (3).

Considering *those in institutions* first, the people who gave us information about these six were two daughters, two sons, and two professionals (a ward sister and a matron of the institution in which the widowed lived). We asked them why the person had entered an institution. Ill health, unsuitable housing, and inability to manage at home – especially with a spouse also in ill health – were the reasons cited for admission:

'Dad looked after her at one time, until it got too much for him. [She had asthma and 'chest complaints'.] It became too much for Dad to look after her and he started to become ill himself. He was in and out of hospital from 1975 onwards.'

'Because the doctor said the house was unfit, so she had to go into a home as she was totally blind, and we had no room at home. It was an old terraced house with no bathroom, cold water, no heating, and an outside toilet.'

Four of the six were mentally confused:

'As far as she's concerned she doesn't know he's dead.'

'She doesn't see you and she doesn't know you.'

All six had difficulty with mobility and/or personal tasks. The four relatives were asked if they ever worried or felt anxious about the widowed. One said 'No':

'It's a great relief now — that's what I feel. A relief that she's well looked after and settled. It's a weight off my mind.'

One felt guilty about the widow being in an old people's home:

'Because I feel a bit guilty because if I'd had the room I'd have her at home, but it's just circumstances. I don't really want her to be in there but she is well looked after.'

But, unlike supporters of the widowed in the community, none of these sons and daughters could see any problems for themselves or their families in the future because of any help or support their widowed parent might need:

'While she's in there we know she's being well looked after. It was a much bigger worry when she was at home.'

'My problem would have been if my mother hadn't been confused and had been left all on her own at home in her eighties and was lonely. I wouldn't have been able to have her here because my mother-in-law's already here and we've no room.'

The four supporters who were *sharing their home* with a widowed person who could not be interviewed were all daughters. The first had a husband and three children. Her father had come to live with them after her mother died as 'he was afraid to be alone'. The daughter had mixed feelings about the wisdom of this move. She described her father's health as 'good' for his age, eighty-three, although he was incontinent. This was one main problem:

'When he passes water he doesn't care where he goes. My bathroom floor and my kitchen floor are constantly flooded. He wees out on the front lawn too — everywhere. . . . It gets on the nerves of the family a lot. He does a lot of tapping with his stick which can be very annoying — I think it's boredom, he never does anything. He needs an interest. As soon as I get up in the morning I have to run around mopping up after him and when I get home from work the first thing I do is run in and mop up after him. He wees everywhere. The other day I caught him doing a wee in one of my pint cups. It's a terrible worry. I never know what I'm going to find.'

When asked how her father felt about sharing a home, the daughter expressed uncertainty:

'I don't know his feelings, he never says if he has any resentments. My husband told him off yesterday for spitting on the carpet and he might resent that − I don't know. Sometimes he uses foul language and my husband has to tell him off about that.'

She did not even know if he missed his wife because he did not communicate with her. One main reason was that he was deaf. He had not been in touch with the health or social services, except to see his doctor about his blood pressure. He also suffered from a number of other physical and mental problems such as rheumatism, sleeplessness, and nerves or depression. The daughter felt no practical problems had emerged for him since the death as she did 'everything' for him. She felt, though, that the doctor should visit him regularly and that loneliness was a problem for him. 'Somewhere to go during the day with people his own age' was one suggestion for helping with this. A downstairs lavatory − which she did not have − was also seen as being helpful with his incontinence, and she expressed a wish for more help from relatives:

'I think if any of my brothers and sisters would come and insist that he went to them for a while it would give me a break. He's been with me now for roughly six or seven months and I feel he should now go for six or seven months to one of the others, but they don't insist strongly enough.'

She felt that caring for her father had adversely affected her life but she seemed resigned to this and felt he would stay with them in their home for the rest of his life:

'If I'm being honest I don't think the home is as happy. The atmosphere is different. . . . It's just something I have to put up with and there's nothing much I can say or do about it.'

The second daughter shared her home with her widowed mother and her husband. Both her parents had moved in with her and her family between one and two years previously because they were both in ill health, with heart conditions. Her mother, the widow, was also mentally confused. The daughter said:

'I can't pursue my life as I did before. I used to go out to work. After my father died it has become impossible to leave the home even for half an hour's shopping. . . . She needs as much looking after as a child. The nurse asks me how long I can go on like this. She seems to think it will wear me down. I think that depends on your temperament. It's a complete tie.'

She felt that it was her responsibility to bear this burden:

'I would do it again − put it like that. I feel they are my responsibility.'

When asked how her mother was feeling about sharing a home the daughter, as in the previous example, felt she could tell us little:

'She doesn't seem to know what the circumstances are. If she could tell you, she would want to be in her own home, but she doesn't communicate. She doesn't seem to know who I am any more.'

The widow could not get about at all, was said to be in 'poor' health for her age, seventy-seven, and suffered from rheumatism, sleeplessness, nerves or depression, irritability, forgetfulness or confusion, and she was blind in one eye. The daughter felt her home was convenient for the widow because 'she only sits in a chair all day and there's a downstairs toilet'.

The daughter described her as totally 'living in the past' and confused, not even realizing her husband was dead:

'She can't even ask for a cup of tea − she doesn't like being looked after and fights me when I take her to the toilet. She is a tall, strong woman still.'

She and her family had not talked to the widow about the possibility of moving although the daughter had thought about this. She said:

'But we are on a boundary and people have had trouble getting people in [to the old people's home]. But we haven't tried − they only take people who are relatively mobile. But I don't think she would want to move to a geriatric place which in our area used to be a workhouse. Now it's impossible to say how she feels.'

The daughter added that it was her 'duty' to care for her mother now. She felt the doctor had done too little for the widow — he had apparently refused to visit her:

> 'She has rigid turns and he [the doctor] told me to put her on the floor and slap her face three times. He has been three times but he's been called since. He just says there is nothing he can do. The nurse asked him to come about her bowel problem [constipation due to prolapse], but again he says there's nothing he can do.'

The daughter shouldered the responsibility for her mother alone — she had a brother but he did not help at all:

> 'My husband thinks I am left to carry the baby — but this happens in every family. My brother is content to leave it to me. Previously we [widow and self] got on very well, we were good friends. That's why I feel I must look after her.'

She felt she herself needed someone to come in and help look after her mother so she could go out more often. When asked about possible problems in the future because of the care she provided, she simply said:

> 'I don't think it *can* get any worse really can it?'

The third daughter who was sharing a home with her father found her time was entirely taken up with caring for him. He had lived with her for four years:

> 'I've never been out for three years. Weight's dropped off me. I'm a skeleton just with the worry. As soon as she [the deceased] went into hospital I couldn't leave Dad.'

Her father, aged eighty-three, was described as 'very confused': 'he's only a cabbage really'. She said he didn't even realize his wife was dead. Sharing her home with the widower had made her 'worn out' and 'mentally strained':

> 'We can't go out and we're stuck in. You can't have any private conversation. I have to bath him and toilet him. I have to do everything for him and keep my eye on him all the time. It's just a full-time job.'

This daughter also saw this caring role as her duty — 'I'll do it while he needs it' — although she realized for the sake of her own health he

should be cared for in an institution. But she said she would not
'dream of sending him anywhere'. She described his health as 'very
poor' for his age, he had a malignant growth in his lung, a heart
condition, and was not at all mobile. At the time of the interview he
was — temporarily the daughter said — in hospital with a broken hip.
He had gone into hospital temporarily to give her the opportunity to
go on holiday and had fallen, broken his hip, and developed pneumonia, whilst there. This gave her a further cause for concern
although the doctor had told her he would not be discharged if he
could not walk:

'I'm worrying about what will happen if he comes home now —
he'll be bedridden.'

The final daughter sharing her home with her widowed father
(aged seventy-six), as well as her husband and two children, said no
problems had emerged from sharing a home:

'I'd rather he was with us than on his own or I'd be worried about
him.'

There were no suggestions that he might move. He had no problems
with mobility and she described his health as 'excellent' for his age —
although he had silicosis and suffered from depression. The daughter
called the doctor 'neglectful' as he 'would never call to see him'. She
added:

'They just don't seem to care about old people.'

This widower apparently did miss his wife and the daughter felt he
had not, and would not, come to terms with the death. Her main
worry about him was his depression:

'When he gets this depression I keep worrying about him.'

Of the nine supporters who were *looking after widowed people but
not living with them*, six were daughters, one was a sister, one a male
friend, and one a female friend. For most of them their involvement
was less than the four we have just described. But one, a female friend
of the widower, visited him several times a day:

'When she'd gone I took over "Pop". I give him all his meals. I come
in and give him his breakfast at 8.15, then at 11 I bring him a
drink. I come in again at 1 with his lunch, then at 4 with his tea,

and at 8 to draw the curtains and put the light on. The last time is
at 10 to give him Horlicks and put him to bed.'

This widower was eighty-three, suffered from chronic bronchitis, and
was 'very deaf'. He was also fairly immobile because of his breathlessness. He had 'bowel problems' which made him incontinent and
suffered from 'occasional depression' and irritability. The supporter
said more help from a district nurse and social worker was needed:

'He could do with a wash down twice a week [instead of once]. I also
asked the social worker if she could arrange for him to go to a
community centre once a week. She said she would arrange it but
I've heard nothing since. I think it would take him out of himself.
He would enjoy it.'

The supporter said she 'carried on' looking after the widower when his
wife had 'left off'. If she did not look after him she said he would have
to go into a home:

'because he doesn't do a thing — just sits all day. . . . It's like
looking after a little baby.'

Although unrelated, she seemed dedicated to her task of looking after
him:

'If there's anything he wants or should have I will always get it for
him. He's part of my life now. . . . What I do I do off my own back.
I knew what I was taking on and I don't care what I do for him.'

His house was described as 'too big for him', he could not do his own
household chores, and he could only live in the bottom part of the
house because he could not get upstairs. However, the respondent
said he would probably stay there for the rest of his life:

'If I have anything to do with it! I'll do all I can possibly manage to
look after him here. . . . They've lived here forty years and brought
their children up here. Pop says he wants to die in the house where
he's always lived.'

Three of these nine supporters said the widowed person might move.
One daughter who lived four-and-a-half-hour's journey away from
her widowed mother said the accommodation was unsuitable:

'She's eight floors up in a high-rise block of flats. She can't always
get out — the lifts are out of order. . . . It's [heating] inadequate
for an old person. There's no heat in the bedroom.'

The widow, who was eighty-two, also had difficulty managing on her own – not through ill health but through loss of interest in life:

> 'She has a lack of interest in cooking. She's not eating, she doesn't bother to cook. We take food down when we go. She doesn't use it. She goes out for bread when the lift is working.'

The daughter wanted the widow to move nearer her and her sister into an old person's bungalow supervised by a warden. No disadvantages were seen in the proposed move:

> 'At the moment if we get a 'phone call what can we do? She's too far away.'

The widow had a number of symptoms – including rheumatism, deafness, sleeplessness, nerves or depression, and forgetfulness or confusion. The daughter felt the doctor had not been helpful enough:

> 'He was not very cooperative. His words were: "What do you want me to do?".'

Another daughter said she and the widow had talked about sharing a home. This widow was aged seventy-two, she had angina and rheumatism, and suffered from sleeplessness, nerves or depression, forgetfulness or confusion, and loss of appetite. Despite these problems, and in part because of them, the daughter was not in favour of the move because the widow would lose her independence, and the daughter would suffer from 'loss of privacy and if she gets too bad I wouldn't be able to have her'. The daughter felt the widow was lonely, however, and needed to meet 'people in a similar position':

> 'I would like to see some sort of counselling service for the bereaved in their homes. . . . She needs someone to talk it all out to and a doctor doesn't have that time.'

The other daughter who said the widow had talked about moving said the widow was aged between 70 and 74, and suffered from 'hardening of the arteries':

> 'She just can't remember what day it is. . . . Oxygen just doesn't get up there.'

She also suffered from arthritis, sleeplessness, irritability, and nerves or depression:

> '"What have I got to live for?" she says.'

The widow was said to miss the deceased a great deal. All the daughter could think of for the widow which might help was a move to a nearby, smaller, flat to get away from the memories. But she added:

'No I don't think there is anything that can be done. She just needs company all the time and you can't have someone there 24 hours a day. The main problem for me is trying to cope with four children, and a business, and trying to be with her at the same time.'

What about the future for these nine supporters? At present seven of them said their lives were being affected by the help and support they were giving the widowed:

'I'm tied down. I can't go out visiting without getting someone to look in and see if he's allright.'

'My life's not my own. I want a job — but not full-time because of my mother.'

'I used to help with a charity group but I don't now. Worry about my mother gives me sleepless nights.'

'I'm getting tired and run down.'

'Life won't be the same again — put it that way.'

Two of the nine said they saw other problems for themselves in the future because of the help and support they gave the widowed, as the widowed person became increasingly dependent.

Discussion

The picture revealed by those who were looking after the widowed who were too ill or too confused to be interviewed themselves gives some indication of the submerged part of the iceberg of need, which has not been identified by the main part of our study. There are also illustrations of the conflicts and strains involved in caring for elderly people at home. Daughters, in particular, start to do more and more things for their parents as they become increasingly frail, confused, and eventually helpless. This is often a gradual process with no sharply defined points of decision. It can develop into an almost intolerable situation imposing enormous psychological and physical demands. A few supporters, including one unrelated person who seemed to be devoting her life to the care of an elderly incontinent widower, apparently need to be needed. Indeed the care given by unrelated people is likely to be seen less as a duty, or a repayment for things the elderly person had done for them in the past, than the care given by daughters and sons. Although few expressed resentment of the elderly person, there was some resentment of other relatives and of professional care givers for not sharing more in the care. It is a situation fraught with potential conflict.

Although one in seven of the people caring for the widows and widowers we interviewed felt their lives had been very restricted by this care, more of them, over a third, envisaged problems in the future. So the problems currently experienced by the restricted supporters, some of which were acute, are likely to hit other supporters at a later stage. Several of the severely restricted were receiving what the familiars felt was inadequate support from medical and social services.

10 What can be done?

One of the reasons for doing this study was that the onset of widowhood is a clearly defined event; in theory it is possible to intervene to help the recently widowed. What has our study revealed about their needs and the ways in which they could be helped?

In this chapter we review some of the things that might be done by statutory and voluntary organizations and by relatives and friends. We start by looking at the views of the widowed people themselves on how they might be helped with one of their main problems – loneliness.

The views of the widowed

The 51% of the widowed who said that loneliness was a problem for them were asked if they felt anything could be done to help with this. The majority, 70%, did not think so. As one put it:

'I think it all boils down to me.'

But some of the negative comments seemed to indicate things that could be done:

'There is nothing to be done. You could go to people, but you can't. On a Sunday nobody goes by. Even a "Good morning" would help. You can't go too often to people.'

'I liked to sew but I'm not interested in anything now. I've no interest in anything – the house needs cleaning. . . . Before I liked

to help anybody but now I feel like nothing. . . . I don't know anything — when someone talks to me, crossing the road I'm not
looking or seeing the cars. That is the nerves, the shock.'

Among the 26% who felt something could be done were those who
wanted supporting services:

'In areas where there are very old people there should be someone
to run round and make contact and check them each night. I have
nobody, I'm quite on my own. So many of your contemporaries are
gone when you live to over ninety.'

Others wanted different housing arrangements:

'If old people could be together, living near, then you could find a
friend to sit with in the evening which would be better.'

And a number wanted friendship:

'By meeting someone genuine. Someone so I could say "I've got a
friend".'

'I'd like to be able to have a friend to visit me. Someone to talk to, to
break the quietness.'

'I don't seem to make friends. It changes when anything's the
matter. What friends you have when you're riding high seem to dis-
appear when you sink to the bottom. People are only interested in
themselves. No one's been to see me.'

Having someone to talk to often seemed particularly important. One
widower who still could not go upstairs where his wife died said:

'I would just like someone to come in here and talk to me.'

The need for companionship emerges clearly in these comments.
Of course the companion most of the widowed want is dead. Most
turn to relatives, friends, and neighbours for help and support in
adjusting to this gap. What can be done to make it possible and easy
for the widowed to maintain these contacts which for many seem to be
lifelines to adjustment and emotional stability, as well as to practical
support and help? And can those with few relatives or friends be
helped to establish new relationships? Some practical possibilities are
considered next.

Some practical needs

These relate to clubs, transport, money, telephones, and housing.

Clubs

Clubs are a possible place to meet new people and can be a source of companionship and support. Some cater specifically for widowed people:

'I think there should be an organization for women — widows — to get people to talk. You need a place to talk troubles over.'

This was a suggestion put forward by one widow we interviewed. There is a such an organization — Cruse — which aims to do this, but only one person in our sample had been in contact with it although two-fifths expressed an interest in its basic activity. Clearly it is unsuccessful in making itself known to many of the people it aims to help. There were branches in or near five of our eight study areas so the problem is not just inadequate geographical cover. We understand that the organization tends to rely on publicity through television documentaries and feature articles in magazines and newspapers to attract its members. But if it is to reach the widowed who are lonely, isolated, and possibly apathetic, a more active approach is needed. Local organizations could identify some of the widowed through death notices in local newspapers although this might give a bias towards the middle class and better off. Alternatively they might approach the registrar of deaths in their areas. This leads to another rather different suggestion: that the marital status of men as well as women should be recorded on the non-confidential part of the death certificate. This would eliminte a sexual inequality as well as enabling widows to be identified at the time of their bereavement.

But many of the widowed were resistant to the idea of meeting others who were bereaved or of going to clubs, and were reluctant to be drawn by relatives and friends into such activities. For others there were financial barriers. Some of the widowed who did not go to clubs, but who would like to, mentioned the expense of going:

'There's the old people's club but you pay 88p for two months to go there — plus the fare to get there. It's so expensive. If you want to go into the bar OAPs must pay 50p to join. Our pensions don't stretch to this. Then there's 5p for a cup of tea.'

There is also the question of transport.

Transport

Transport is needed if the elderly widowed are to maintain contact with relatives and friends, to go to clubs, or to pursue a range of other activities. We have shown that 22% have difficulty or cannot use public transport. A quarter of the widowed had been deprived of private transport on their widowhood. Cheap bus-passes, possessed by two-thirds, may be a boon to those who can use buses. Certainly those who went to clubs were more likely to have a cheap bus-pass than those who did not do so, 70% compared with 42%. But the fact that so many cannot use public transport, or only with difficulty, and the inadequacy of such services in many areas, mean that it is difficult for many of the elderly widowed to go and see relatives and friends when they would like to do so. They become dependent on relatives and friends coming to see them. This pushes them into a more passive role in their relationships as they are less able to initiate contacts. Feelings of dependency are therefore accentuated at a time when they need help and encouragement in establishing independence. Volunteers might be prepared to drive the disabled and frail widowed to see relatives, and some of the elderly widowed who have and drive cars themselves, 13%, might well be willing to help with this. But they would need a travel allowance. As one widow said, it is expensive 'to get about, you can't afford it now'. And another said if she had more money she would 'probably get about a bit more, but you've got to think twice about the petrol now'.

Money

It takes money to keep in touch with friends and relatives, to make new contacts, and to engage in activities ensuring frequent social interaction. We have shown that those who felt they were short of money had greater problems with loneliness and more difficulty in adjusting to the death of their spouse.

An analysis of the sources of income for those who said they found money a problem with those who did not shows that those who had a

pension other than an ordinary old-age one were comparatively unlikely to find money a problem: 20% of them compared with 36% of
those without such a pension; whereas for those receiving supplementary benefit the position was reversed, 42% found money a problem, against 25%. Part of, but not all, the financial problems of the
widowed were related to a deterioration in their financial position
since their spouse died. Just over half said they were now worse off
financially and one in six were 'a great deal worse off'. Delays in
receiving benefits, experienced by about one in ten, added to their
financial problems and created anxieties and uncertainty.

The middle class were as likely as the working class to be facing a
fall in their income, but they were less likely to find money a problem,
partly, at any rate, because more of them had a retirement pension in
addition to their old-age one. More money, particularly for the
working-class widowed, could help them adjust to their situation and
relieve some of the real hardships experienced.

An illustration of some of the effects of being short of money is
given by a widow receiving just a widow's pension and some help from
relatives. She went short of 'clothes, shoes, and all sorts of things'. She
also had a cheap bus-pass but said:

> 'it costs 20p each time to go to the doctor or clinic — appointments
> are after cheaper fares finish.'

She had broken her reading glasses and said she 'could not pay for any
more out of £19 per week'. The funeral had cost over £200:

> '£20 (funeral expenses) is ridiculous — that's what you get. I had a
> letter from the social security to go and see them but I wasn't able to
> go because of my foot.'

When asked about clubs and societies, she commented:

> 'You haven't much money to go anywhere on £19.

The telephone

The telephone is a way of keeping in touch with people. But again it
costs money. Forty per cent of the widowed lived in households
without a telephone and this proportion was similar for those who
lived alone and those who lived with others. As expected there was a
clear trend with social class: the proportion with a telephone fell

from 85% of those in Social Class I to 44% of those in Social Class V.
And associated with this, 73% of those who owned their home had a
telephone, compared with 49% of those in council houses or flats, and
42% of those in privately rented accommodation.

Naturally, those who had a telephone in their home were more
likely to use it regularly than those who had to use a call box or go to
neighbours. But 43% of those without a telephone said they sometimes spoke to relatives and friends on the telephone, including 17%
who did so at least weekly. Among those with a telephone, the proportion using it to talk to relatives, friends, or neighbours at least
weekly was three-quarters, including a quarter who used it daily.

Those who were physically handicapped were no more or less likely
to have a telephone than those who were not, but those in poor health
were *less* likely to have a telephone than those who rated their health
as excellent, good, or fair, 37% against 63%.

Possession of a telephone was not related to the age of the widowed
but the older widowed were less likely to speak on the telephone than
younger ones: 22% of those aged under 75 never spoke on the 'phone
in comparison with 36% of those 75 and over.

The telephone seemed to be used to augment rather than substitute
for face-to-face contacts as no differences were found between speaking on the telephone and frequency of personal contacts with relatives
and friends. Nor did possession of, or speaking on, the telephone
relate to emotional adjustment or perceptions of loneliness as a problem, although some of the widowed commented on the importance of
a telephone to them:

'That's my lifeline, the bills worry me though.'

But the telephone is not only a means of keeping in touch with
relatives and friends, it is a potential lifeline in an emergency, giving a
sense of security to those now living alone − although, as we have just
shown, those living alone were no more likely to have a telephone than
those who lived with others, and it was those in poor health who were
least likely to have one. Only 2% of those in our study received
financial help from social services towards a telephone. In our view
such grants should be more generally available.

Housing

This study has shown the considerable attachment of elderly widowed
people to their homes despite some of the practical disadvantages.

The elderly widowed for the most part want to retain their indepen-dence, to stay in their own home, and to be near relatives and friends. Conflicts arise when stairs or inadequate facilities make it impractical for elderly frail widows or widowers to stay in their home and retain their independence, and a solution might seem to be to move in with relatives. Policies which encourage improvements, modifications, and sometimes the division of existing homes may sometimes resolve such conflicts. Adaptations such as ramps, bath aids, kitchen aids, heating assistance, and upgrading of accommodation, as well as tele-phones and alarm systems are eligible, in theory, for consideration under improvement or other local authority grants schemes. In practice, however, waiting lists may be long, funds inadequate, and the help needed to install equipment and give instruction on usage may not be available. If such changes could be arranged more readily this might enable more elderly widowed people to stay in their home rather than face the upheaval of a move and the loss of independence. There is still the hassle of arranging and supervising such changes, and indeed of organizing the upkeep of a home for the elderly who live alone. The 'gifted housing' scheme of Help the Aged in which they are prepared to convert, improve, and maintain homes which are too big for elderly people and suitable to conversion into separate homes may help those with such houses. Eighty-four per cent of the widowed who lived alone had four or more rooms in their homes. Could not the scheme be extended to cover the maintenance and im-provement of smaller homes which cannot be converted? This might be acceptable to the widowed who are childless. Those with children may want to retain something to leave to their children when they die.

Another type of conflict arises when widowed people are faced with a choice between a home with valued memories and good neighbours but far away from relatives, and a new home with no known friends or neighbours but a particular and important relative nearby. This type of conflict can never be completely avoided but housing authorities should be encouraged to make deliberate efforts to keep extended families together and to house young people near to their parents when they want it.

While appropriate housing, clubs, telephones for the frail and those living on their own, more transport facilities, and particularly more money might resolve some of the problems facing the elderly widowed, they do have other needs. How can relatives and friends help or hinder in their attempts to comfort the elderly widowed and assist their adjustment?

Actions and attitudes of relatives and friends

Parkes (1972) has said that one of the major problems of adjusting to bereavement is that the bereaved are not permitted to express their grief in company. Lopata (1973) found that the widows in her sample often reported being shunned by friends as they felt uncomfortable in the widow's presence. Some people do not know how to approach the bereaved, they do not know what to say and become embarrassed. Death is a taboo subject. The widowed may be avoided in an attempt to ignore it and thus they may become even more isolated and lonely. Some comments of the widowed in our study illustrate these problems:

'You still feel on your own (even though I live with the family). There can be a roomful of people, nobody seems to want to bother with you. They're frightened of saying his name.'

'People just don't ask do they?'

'They won't mention his name.'

'People round here don't want to talk about it. They are hard. They say "Don't cry", but I can't stop crying.'

'When you're a widow and you start talking about it they're not interested. That's why I've not cried, I've just been a frozen thing. People turn away if you tell them your troubles.'

One widow said that her daughter and her sister were too involved in their own problems to consider hers. She said she didn't feel able to talk to anyone, her family 'did not confide' in each other. As a result she said:

'I feel as though I'm locked and if it breaks I shall make a fool of myself.'

A familiar said she was 'fed up' with the widow concentrating on the past:

'All the time she surrounds herself with it [the past]. I get fed up with it all. I go there to try to cheer her up and she just goes on and on about the past.'

Avoidance may worsen any feelings of social isolation and interfere with adjustment. Who did the widowed feel it was best to talk to about their feelings when someone dies? When asked, most, 65%, mentioned a relative; 19% a close friend, 3% a doctor, and 3% a clergyman. Over three-quarters, 79%, had found a relative most helpful and 20% found friends and neighbours to be of most help in this sense. In addition, 3% mentioned a general practitioner and 1% a clergyman. Four per cent said they found no one helpful. A comment from one who looked outside her network of relatives and friends for this sort of help was:

> 'If a social worker or somebody could come to have a chat with you. It's like cutting off your right arm in a way. If somebody could tell you "You'll get over it".'

What part did and could general practitioners, social workers, and other social services play in helping the elderly widowed? The role of the general practitioner is discussed first.

The role of the general practitioner

Although the general practitioner was the professional person the widowed were most likely to have been in contact with since their bereavement, just under a quarter of the elderly widowed had been visited by a general practitioner after their spouse died but before the funeral. Two-fifths of the doctors thought that elderly people should be visited at home when they were widowed and most doctors thought this should be done as soon as possible, but, even when doctors felt this was the right thing to do, less than half of their elderly widowed patients had such a visit. Does this matter? For the most part general practice is based on self-referral by patients initially. On the whole this seems to work reasonably well, but a study by Williamson and his colleagues (1964) indicated that the system of self-reporting of illness failed to meet the needs of old people. And when an elderly person loses their husband or wife the feelings of helplessness and hopelessness associated with bereavement may make it difficult for them to recognize their needs in the first place or to do anything about it if they are aware of such needs. Depression is often associated with apathy and nearly half the elderly widowed said they had problems with nerves or depression — and for almost three-quarters of these the problem had developed since, or been accentuated by, the death of their spouse. If, in addition, they had looked to their husband or wife for advice about whether or when to consult a doctor, they will now be missing this spur. In practice, 16% of those reporting nerves or depression had had no contact with a general practitioner since their spouse died.

In addition to the emotional barriers of indifference and inertia that may inhibit the elderly widowed from consulting their doctors there were, for a sizeable minority, the practical problems of immobility: 5% could not go out on their own and a further 11% could only do so with difficulty.

So if most general practitioners are unwilling to take the initiative and either contact their elderly widowed patients themselves or arrange for an appropriate member of their team to do so, there is a real danger that the most vulnerable will not get the help they need. Those who are isolated – physically, emotionally, of socially – will not be identified. In consequence their problem will become intensified. One form of isolation is likely to lead to another: the physically isolated may accept their situation passively and drift into social isolation or excessive dependence on a single relative, friend, or neighbour, if one is available; the emotionally isolated may cut themselves off from relatives or friends who might help. A vicious circle will accentuate difficulties to a point where they may become irreversible.

It seems to us that to look after elderly widowed patients effectively demands personal care, family care, home care, and continuity of care: four fundamental and distinguishing aspects of general practice. And we would therefore expect general practitioners who are concerned to give this type of care to visit the homes of all their patients when they are widowed – or to be in contact with a social worker or nurse, known to the widowed, who has done so.

Our recommendation that all widowed people should be visited stems, in part, from our belief that when people are widowed it is not only helpful for them to have the support of people who care but also that they need to re-define and establish their relationship with people who are meaningful to them. In our view the relationship that general practitioners have with their elderly patients should be important enough to need this recognition and emphasis. We feel that contact at this time is not only important for the future relationship but can also provide insights and clues about the bereaved's situation and needs. It also gives an opportunity to talk to the widowed about the care that was given to the spouse who died, to find out about any anxieties or guilt feeling that they have, and to give reassurance. This reassurance is even more important in view of the finding that, while a certain amount of anger and guilt are a typical component of the early stages of grief, Parkes (1965) found that ideas of guilt and self-reproach were greatest in bereaved people who subsequently develop a psychiatric illness. This is partly supported by the finding in the present study that those widows and widowers who wished that something had been done differently adjusted worse emotionally.

Other studies (e.g. Raphael 1977) have demonstrated the effectiveness of supportive intervention to high-risk widows and widowers. Home visits are likely to assist the general practitioner to identify those in need of help. If the widow or widower has no supportive network of relatives or friends, referral to counselling services may help (Parkes 1980).

Another suggestion about the role of the general practitioner in helping the elderly widowed relates to the prescription of minor tranquillizers, sedatives, and hypnotics. Our findings suggest a tendency to prescribe pills rather give supportive care to the bereaved. At the same time there is anxiety among many elderly widowed about becoming dependent on drugs, and a reluctance to take drugs. Possibly they feel that the process of grieving may be protracted rather than helped by drugs. Another danger identified by our study is that general practitioners are not always aware of the prescribed drugs that their patients are taking, so there is a possibility of interaction and side effects. It may take more time and effort to sit in sympathy and listen than to prescribe pills, but it would seem that elderly widowed patients are more likely to need and to appreciate the sympathetic listening.

Thirdly we would point out that the ability of general practitioners to help their elderly patients when they are widowed depends on the relationship that has been built up over time and particularly on the care given during the terminal illness. Doctors who visited relatively frequently during this time and those who were willing to discuss the situation and probable outcome with the prospective widow or widower were more able to give comfort and support in bereavement. Over this period continuity of care is probably particularly important.

A fourth suggestion is for more emphasis on coping with dying, with death, and with bereavement at all stages of medical education: undergraduate, postgraduate, and in further education. It has been

224   Life After A Death

calculated (Cartwright, Hockey, and Anderson 1973:79) that between a quarter and three-tenths of hospital-bed days are taken up by people who will be dead within twelve months, but only 4% of people dying in an institution in 1969 died in a teaching hospital (and fewer still, less than 1%, in a hospital or institution specializing in terminal care). So medical students get inadequate experience and training in dealing with a common, indeed universal, problem. Yet it is a situation which imposes emotional demands. Doctors need support and understanding to be able to respond to it adequately.

The role of social and voluntary services

Apart from the general practitioner the other professionals and social services who had been to the homes of the widowed are shown in *Table 72*. Nearly half had been visited by a vicar, priest, or rabbi and most of those who had been visited found the visit helpful, although one in ten had not done so. There was no significant difference between the various religious groups in the proportion receiving such a visit but more of those who said they had a belief, philosophy, or practice that they felt had helped them adjust to or accept their widowhood had been visited, 58% compared with 39% of those

Table 72   Visits from social and other services

	Proportion of widowed visited
	%
District nurse	14
Health visitor	10
Other nurse	2
Social worker	13
Someone from social security	27
Someone about insurance	29
Vicar, priest, or rabbi	48
Voluntary organization worker	3
Home help	16
Mobile library	5
Other official person – identified	5
Someone, uncertain of identity	–
None of these	19
Number of widowed (= 100%)	349

without such a belief. And those who had been visited by a vicar, priest, or rabbi scored rather better than the others on our adjustment scale with an average of 3.6 against 3.2 for the others. It may be recalled that having a belief or philosophy did not appear to be related to adjustment. Possibly vicars and priests are more likely to visit those who are socially integrated? They had visited 46% of those living alone compared with 53% of those living with others − a difference which might have arisen by chance. More significantly they had seen 50% of those who saw some one person more than once a week, but only 32% of the isolated who did not see anybody so regularly. If vicars and priests made a point of identifying and visiting the elderly widowed, this might be helpful. Again it could be made easier for them to do this in a systematic way in an area if the marital status of men who die was recorded on the public part of death certificates.

The 'insurance man' was the next most common visitor (see also Hunt 1978) and again most (nine out of ten) of the widowed had found him helpful. They were less appreciative of visits from someone from social security and from social workers. For both of these, one in five of those who had been visited said the person had not been helpful.

Few of the widowed, 14%, said they would have liked one or more of the people listed in *Table 72* to visit, but it was a social worker who was most often mentioned, by 4% of all the widowed. Comments about why they would have liked a social worker to call were for the most part vague or related to money and companionship:

'Just to find out about everything − about the money. Just because I've got that little bit of pension I can't have anything else.'

'In the hospital they told me one would come so I expected one to come and no one came. I was allright but they could have come the once I thought.'

'Just for a bit of company really.'

'I would have liked to ask her about my tax problems.'

Social workers were no more or less likely to have visited the widowed who lived alone, or the isolated, than those who lived with others or saw people fairly frequently.

In previous chapters we have shown that the disabled widowed relied mainly on relatives, friends, and neighbours for help and that more of the widowed had meals brought in by relatives, friends, and neighbours than got them through meals on wheels or a luncheon club. Few others felt they wanted meals on wheels. More common needs were for jobs and other meaningful activities, and it is towards helping the elderly widowed to obtain these that the social agencies might direct particular attention.

Nineteen per cent of the widowed said they would like a job now; all but two of these said part-time work would be preferred. But as one widower put it:

'I would like to do more work to [help me] forget, but in a village you can't get more work.'

Over a third of all the widowed said they had not been in a position to help any of their relatives, friends, or neighbours since their spouse died, but would like to do so. Voluntary visiting of hospital patients was often mentioned as a possibility. Perhaps hospitals and good neighbouring schemes could be more aware, and encouraging, of such potential help:

'I'm looking after people more lonely than myself. That's my advice, go out and find somebody more lonely than yourself. Forget your sorrows and loneliness. Find something to do. I worked that out for myself when I found I was sitting around moping.'

Self-help and other voluntary groups may be able to work out ways of matching needs and sources of help possibly by going across the boundaries of such different groups as widows and single-parent families as Robinson (1981) has suggested. So Cruse and Gingerbread may have much to offer each other.

Summing-up

The widowed need to adjust to their new state while preoccupied with the painful struggle to master their grief. What can be done to help? One important thing is to let them grieve. In our present society, mourning ceremonies have become mostly perfunctory and possibly this had made us all, relatives, friends, neighbours, doctors, social workers, and vicars, less sensitive to the need for the fundamental and often prolonged process of grieving. People need support while they are grieving, with opportunities to describe their feelings and to talk about the person who has died. They may also need opportunities to be alone. Grieving is not done all at once; it is an intermittent process of varying intensity and with frequent relapses. The bereaved need time, patience, and understanding. Some may be helped by pills but more patients are reluctant to start taking drugs than doctors seem to realize (Cartwright in press). All the bereaved need sympathy; pills are no substitute even though some doctors seem to use them in this way.

Another need is for help with the practicalities of their day-to-day lives. Many have to adjust to living alone. Widowers may have to shop and cook for the first time in their lives, while widows are likely to have to adjust to shopping and cooking for one. In their new lives they need to find a purpose and meaningful activities – but what is acceptable and stimulating for one may be depressing and unhelpful for another. The widowed, like others, differ widely in their needs and desire for company, for solitude, and for all types of activity.

In addition to the loneliness of missing a particular companion, the difficulties of adjusting to a new and often restricted life situation, and the pain of coping with grief, the widowed in our study faced the common problems of the elderly: ill health and disability with their restrictions on activity; dealing with inconvenient but treasured homes; maintaining contact with valued relatives and friends; and coping with all these problems on a reduced and declining budget.

There is the danger that in this time of financial stringency some of our suggestions about clubs, housing, telephones, transport, and money, will be perceived as incurring increased and unacceptable costs. To save some of these 'costs' would be a false economy. Telephones for the frail and elderly who live alone may give the elderly persons themselves the confidence to continue living in the community and enable their relatives and friends to provide the contact and support needed. Similar 'economies' may be achieved by improvements and adaptations to homes, so that elderly people do not have to cope with awkward stairs between their bedroom and the lavatory or commit themselves to enormous fuel bills in order to maintain a reasonable temperature. In these sorts of ways the cost of institutional care may sometimes be saved at the same time as the quality of life is enhanced.

However institutional care cannot always be avoided. The information from this study and others (see Isaacs, Livingstone, and Neville 1972 and Cartwright, Hockey, and Anderson 1973) about the way wives and husbands care for their dying spouses and the readiness of daughters and other relatives to support the elderly widowed suggest that our society may already be imposing an unreasonable burden on relatives who are willing but frail, and creating intolerable conflicts for dutiful and caring daughters who are also mothers and wage earners. The fact that admission to an institution, even for those in need of permanent care, so often involves sharing a room, relinquishing almost all possessions, and forgoing privacy and even dignity, adds to the burden of decision and can create guilt and despondency.

Some of the other needs we have identified for transport, housing maintenance, and schemes to involve the widowed in meaningful activities might be taken up by voluntary associations; and links between self-help groups with matching needs and resources could be fruitful. But the present emphasis on voluntary work is in danger of creating cynicism. And voluntary groups need encouragement and financial support.

There is also a need for money in a more direct form. We have shown how problems of loneliness and difficulties in adjusting to a new role are exacerbated by lack of money. And this study was done more than two years ago, before major cuts in health, social, and transport services. These will make it more difficult for elderly people to see their relatives and friends, to obtain grants for house improvements, to get to hospital when they need care, to be supported by a home help when they become more disabled, to obtain sheltered housing when they need some supervision, or to be admitted to an appropriate institution when the support of relatives, friends, and neighbours can no longer enable them to lead a reasonable life in the community. Our study has shown the large part played by the informal network of relatives, friends, and neighbours in sustaining the elderly widowed. They too need support if they are not to be overburdened by the demands put on them.

Finally, there is the problem of identifying and then helping the depressed, apathetic, and isolated widows and widowers who may well be under-represented in our sample. Informal networks of neighbours, vicars and priests, voluntary organizations for helping the widowed and the elderly, social workers, and community health workers, all have a part to play in this but we have argued that general practitioners have a particular responsibility here and that they should be encouraged and stimulated to perform this role more adequately than they do at present. A basic need is to help this widower and others like him:

'I'm going to go outside this winter and sit for two hours until my temperature drops − I know all about hypothermia − then I shall just die.'

Appendix I
Selection of the study areas

The study of the elderly widowed was carried out in eight areas in England. The areas were registration districts or combinations of registration districts selected with a probability proportional to the number of deaths after stratification by area. To select the eight registration districts, the total number of deaths registered in England during 1978 were summed for each metropolitan and non-metropolitan county. Starting with London and the metropolitan counties, the counties were then listed in geographical order from North to South, and the number of deaths were summed cumulatively. The total number of deaths (550,063) was divided by eight to give the sampling interval (68,758), and a number under this was selected from a book of random numbers to give a random starting point (19,815). The area which contained this number was taken as the first study area. The other areas were obtained by successive additions of the sampling fraction to the starting point. Within the chosen counties a detailed breakdown of deaths occurring in 1978 for each of the registration districts was obtained from the Office of Population Censuses and Surveys. When necessary, the registration districts were grouped together geographically so that each district or combination of districts had at least 2,400 deaths registered during the year. This ensured that at least 200 deaths each month were likely to occur in each district. The districts were then listed from North to South, summed cumulatively, and the areas containing the sampling points identified. The areas selected are shown in *Table A*.

Table A Study districts

	County	Region	Total number of deaths in 1978	
			In county	In district(s)
District(s):				
Havering	Greater London	London	84,568	3,404
North Tyneside West ⎫ Newcastle-upon-Tyne ⎭	Tyne and Wear	North Eastern	15,384	5,815
Solihull North ⎫ Solihull South ⎬ Coventry ⎭	West Midlands	Midland	30,582	4,695
High Peak ⎫ Bakewell ⎬ Chesterfield ⎭	Derbyshire	Northern	9,752	4,178
North Warwickshire Nuneaton Rugby Warwick and Leamington Stratford-on-Avon Southam Alcester Shipston-on-Stour	Warwickshire	Midland	4,719	4,719*
Wigan ⎫ Leigh ⎭	Greater Manchester	North Western	33,958	3,682
Bristol	Avon	Western	11,507	6,783
Barnstaple Bideford Holsworthy Okehampton Tiverton	Devon	South Western	13,485	2,701

* All districts in Warwickshire were taken to ensure the sample size was sufficient.

Appendix II
The rationale of the sample

Ideally we would have liked a sample of widows and widowers over a certain age. But the marital status of men who die is not recorded on the non-confidential part of the death certificate. In addition, the age of the surviving widow or widower is only on the confidential part of the death certificate. So to cover a complete sample of widows and widowers of a particular age, we would have had to start from a sample of deaths of all men and of all married women whatever their ages. This would have been impractical since so many would have been ineligible for inclusion in the final study.

Table B   Effects of different sampling strategies

	Base deaths of married people aged 65 or more			Base deaths of married men aged 65 or more and married women aged 60 or more		
	Widowers	*Widows*	*Both sexes*	*Widowers*	*Widows*	*Both sexes*
Proportion of widows and widowers:						
Aged 65 or more *not* included	12.2%	3.6%	6.6%	2.8%	3.6%	3.3%
Aged 60 or more *not* included	23.4%	12.3%	15.9%	15.8%	12.3%	13.4%
Proportion included aged:						
Under 50	0.2%	0.8%	0.7%	0.3%	0.8%	0.7%
50–54	0.4%	1.8%	1.4%	0.7%	1.8%	1.5%
55–59	1.0%	4.5%	3.5%	2.6%	4.5%	3.9%
60–64	4.8%	14.3%	11.6%	11.8%	14.3%	13.5%
Total under 60	1.6%	7.1%	5.6%	3.6%	7.1%	6.1%
Total under 65	6.4%	21.4%	17.2%	15.4%	21.4%	19.6%
Estimated sex distribution of widows and widowers	28.3%	71.7%	100.0%	32.6%	67.4%	100.0%

Source: Office of Population Censuses and Surveys (1978) *Marriage and divorce statistics 1975.*

At the pilot stage we considered the effects of different sampling strategies. In any event we would have to ascertain for the men who died whether or not they had been married at the time. But if we took different age cut-offs for the deaths, how many elderly widows and widowers would be excluded, how many younger widows and widowers would be included initially, and what would be the sex ratio among our final sample? The data to answer these three questions are in *Table B* for two different sampling strategies, one starting from a sample of deaths of married people aged 65 or more, and the other from the deaths of married men aged 65 or more and women aged 60 or more.

We thought the most important principle was to minimize the proportion of the elderly widowed aged 65 or more not covered by the sample. If we had taken a sample of deaths of all married people aged 65 or more, one in eight of elderly widowers would have been excluded from the sample, because on average men are older than their wives.

Taking a different age cut-off for the deaths of married men and women not only led to a more comprehensive sample of elderly widowed people but also improved the sex ratio of the sample. It meant that rather more younger widowers were included but the proportion under sixty was still small, 4%, and we decided not to exclude them. This means that the sampling frame is straightforward even though it is not precisely what we would have liked.

Appendix III
Statistical significance and sampling errors

There are a number of factors, particularly the nature of the data and the stage at which precise hypotheses are often formulated, which violate some of the conditions in which statistical tests of significance apply and thus make interpretation difficult. For this reason they are rarely referred to in the text, in an attempt to avoid the appearance of spurious precision which the presentation of such tests might seem to imply. But in the absence of more satisfactory techniques these tests have been used to give some indication of the probability of differences occurring by chance.

Chi-square and chi-square trend tests have been applied constantly when looking at the data from this survey. Correlations, t-tests, and tests of differences in proportions have also been used. These tests have influenced decisions about what differences to present and how much verbal 'weight' to attach to them. In general, attention has not been drawn to any difference which statistical tests suggest might have occurred by chance five or more times in 100.

Another difficulty about presenting results from a study like this with almost 300 items of basic information is that of selection. Inevitably not all cross-analyses are carried out – about 2,000 for the whole study – and only a fraction of these are presented, which of course gives rise to difficulty in interpreting significance. Positive results are more often given than negative ones. Readers may sometimes wonder why certain further analyses are not reported. In many cases – but not all – the analysis will have been done but the result found to be negative or inconclusive.

Table C shows the sampling errors for a number of characteristics. Their calculation is based on observed variations in the eight study areas (for the appropriate formula see Gray and Corlett 1950). In no instance was the design effect more than 1.3.

Table C Sampling errors

	Mean proportion	Range in the eight study areas	Sampling error	Estimated random sampling error*	Mean ± two sampling errors	Design effect**
Proportion of widow(er)s saying loneliness is a problem	51%	43%–59%	2.1%	2.5%	47%–55%	0.8
Proportion of widow(er)s not come to terms with death	28%	17%–36%	2.5%	2.3%	24%–34%	1.1
Proportion of widow(er)s not looking forward	66%	55%–78%	3.0%	2.4%	60%–72%	1.3
Proportion of widow(er)s wishing something done differently before death	23%	9%–34%	2.8%	2.1%	17%–29%	1.3
Proportion of widow(er)s who see children daily	31%	25%–40%	2.1%	2.3%	27%–35%	0.9
Proportion of widow(er)s who said death expected	40%	29%–53%	2.9%	2.4%	31%–49%	1.2
Proportion of widow(er)s living alone	78%	69%–89%	2.3%	2.0%	72%–84%	1.2
Proportion of widow(er)s saying money was a problem	29%	17%–39%	2.9%	2.3%	23%–35%	1.3
Proportion of widow(er)s in poor health	8%	2%–15%	1.5%	1.3%	5%–11%	1.2
Proportion of widow(er)s taking psychotropic drugs	37%	26%–52%	3.1%	2.5%	29%–45%	1.3
Proportion of cancer deaths	22%	17%–30%	1.7%	2.1%	19%–25%	0.8

* If a random sample throughout the country, that is, $\left\{ \dfrac{p\,(1-p)}{n} \left(1 - \dfrac{n}{N}\right) \right\}^{\frac{1}{2}}$

** The ratio of the sampling error with the given two-stage sample design to the estimated random sampling error.

Appendix IV
Classification of social class

The last full-time occupation of a deceased man is recorded on the death certificate, the previous occupation if he had retired, and the husband's occupation if the deceased was a married woman. The occupation was classified according to the Registrar General's Classification of Occupations (1970) into six groups — five social classes distinguished by the Registrar General, with Social Class III, skilled occupations, subdivided into non-manual and manual.

At the interview information was collected about the deceased's main job, if male, or about the respondent's main occupation if the deceased was female. As the sample is based on people over retirement age it is possible that some bias may be involved as, for most, the question was retrospective. The occupations obtained at the interview were coded in the same way as those recorded on the death certificate.

Table D compares the social-class distribution of the deceased's or widower's

Table D   Social class — distributions

	Interview	Death certificate
Social class:	%	%
I Professional	3	1
II Intermediate	17	14
III Skilled		
Non-manual	9	11
Manual	48	46
IV Partly skilled	16	19
V Unskilled	7	9
Number of deaths for which information available (= 100%)	339	358

main occupation from the interview with that of the occupation on the death certificate. A cross-analysis of data from the death certificates and the interviews showed that 63% were in precisely the same category, 19% differed by one category, and 18% by more than one. The differences were in both directions and fairly evenly balanced. A cross-analysis was done for men and women separately. This showed complete agreement for 63% of the widows, while 21% differed by one category, and 16% by more than one. Agreement for widowers was less good. A similar proportion, 62%, agreed completely but fewer, 12%, were one category different and more, 26%, differed by more than one category.

In the report, data from the death certificate were used. Social class could be classified from the information there for 99% of the deaths. In 1% the occupation given was armed forces or the description of occupation seemed inadequate.

Appendix V
Classification of cause of death

The underlying cause of death had been classified by the Office of Population Censuses and Surveys into the four-digit International Classification of Causes of Death (ninth revision). We grouped these in the way shown in *Table E* which also gives the distribution among our sample. Response rates were unrelated to the cause of death.

Table E Classification of cause of death

	ICD number	Sample selected	Sample interviewed	Response rate
Underlying cause:				
Malignant neoplasms	140−208	112	81	72%
Other neoplasms	210−239	0	0	
Ischaemic heart disease	410−414	158	114	72%
Cerebrovascular accident	430−438	53	39	74%
Other diseases of the circulatory system	390−405, 415−429, 440−459	42	33	79%
Pneumonia and influenza	480−487	46	35	76%
Chronic obstructive pulmonary disease and allied conditions*	490−496	36	28	78%
Other diseases of the respiratory system	460−478, 500−519	5	4	***
Psychoses	290−299	1	1	***
Accidents, poisonings, violence	800−999	5	5	***
Other	**	28	21	75%
Total		486	361	74%

* Bronchitis unspec., chronic bronchitis, emphysema, asthma, extrinsic allergic alveolitis, and chronic airways obstruction NOS.
** 000−136, 300−389, 520−799.
*** Inadequate numbers.

Appendix VI
Classification of drugs

This classification was based on the DHSS Drug Master Index — the 'Straight alpha version' (DHSS 1978). The division into minor and major tranquillizers was made on the basis of Peter Parish's classification (Parish 1976) and the grouping was suggested by Jasper Woodcock from the Institute for the Study of Drug Dependence. The way this was done is shown in *Table F* alongside the distribution of all prescribed medicines reported by our sample.

Table F   Classification of drugs

	Drug Master Index codes	Number
Psychotropic drugs		
Anti-depressant or stimulant (including combinations of these)	02−2,3,4	14
Minor tranquillizers	01−2,3	131
Major tranquillizers	01−3	10
Anti-depressant and sedative/tranquillizer combinations	02−5	4
Appetite suppressant (Non-CNS stimulants)	02−7	2
Other preparations acting on the nervous system }	01−1,4,6,7,8,9 02−1,6,8	47
Preparations acting on the gastro-intestinal system	03	50
Preparations acting on the cardiovascular system and diuretics	04	154
Preparations acting on the respiratory system or affecting allergic reactions }	05 13	30
Preparations prescribed for rheumatism	06	49
Preparations acting systemically on infections	08	31
Preparations with hormone or anti-hormone activity	09	16
Preparations affecting nutrition or blood	10,12	22
Preparations acting locally on skin and mucous membrane or acting on the eye }	14 15	28
Other prescribed medicines }	07,11,16,17, 18,19	5
Inadequate, name of preparation unknown		61
Total	−	654

Appendix VII
Classification of conditions

Conditions for which prescribed medicines had been taken were classified according to the International Classification of Diseases 1975, then grouped in the way shown in *Table G*, alongside the distribution.

Table G   Classification of conditions

Conditions	ICD number	Number
Infective and parasitic	001–136	10
Neoplasms	140–239	0
Endocrine, nutritional, and metabolic diseases and symptoms	240–279, 783	24
Diseases of the blood and blood forming organs	280–289	10
Diseases and symptoms of the circulatory system	390–485, 785	111
Bronchitis	466, 490, 491	10
Other diseases and symptoms of the respiratory system	} 460–519 (except 466, 490–1), 787	49
Diseases of the digestive system and symptoms of the gastro-intestinal tract	520–577, 787	45
Diseases and symptoms of the genito-urinary system	580–629, 788	27
Diseases of the skin and subcutaneous tissue	680–709, 782	19
Diseases of the musculo and skeletal system and symptoms referable to the limb and joints	710–739, 781	90
Congenital abnormalities	740–759	0
Mental disorders, nervousness, and debility	290–319, 799	175
·Including nerves or depression		(60)
Including sleeplessness		(86)
Diseases and symptoms of the nervous system and sense organs	320–389, 781	14
Other symptoms, senility, and ill-defined conditions	780, 784, 789–797	45
Inadequate		25
Total		654

References

AGE CONCERN (1974) *The Attitudes of the Retired and the Elderly.* London: National Old People's Welfare Council.

ANDERSON, R. (1980a) Prescribed Medicines: Who Takes What? *Journal of Epidemiology and Community Health* **34**: 299–304.

—— (1980b) The Use of Repeatedly Prescribed Medicines. *Journal of the Royal College of General Practitioners* **30**: 609–13.

ARCAND, R. and WILLIAMSON, J. (1981) An Evaluation of Home Visiting of Patients by Physicians in Geriatric Medicine. *British Medical Journal* **283**: 718–20.

BERKMAN, L. K. and SYME, S. L. (1979) Social Networks, Host Resistance and Mortality: A Nine-Year Follow-up Study of Alameda County Residents. *American Journal of Epidemiology* **109**: 186–204.

BLAU, Z. (1961) Structural Constraints on Friendships in Old Age. *American Sociological Review* **26** (June): 429–39.

—— (1973) *Old Age in a Changing Society.* New York: Franklin Watts.

BOWLBY, J. (1960) Grief and Mourning in Infancy and Early Childhood. *The Psychoanalytic Study of the Child* **15**: 9–63.

BOWLING, A. (in draft) Caring for the Elderly Widowed — The Burden on Their Supporters.

BUCHAN, I. C. and RICHARDSON, I. M. (1973) *Time Study of Consultations in General Practice. (Scottish Health Studies No. 27.)* Scottish Home & Health Department.

CARTWRIGHT, A. (1963) Memory Errors in a Morbidity Survey. *Milbank Memorial Fund Quarterly* **41**: 5–24.

—— (1967) *Patients and Their Doctors.* London: Routledge and Kegan Paul.

—— (1979) *The Dignity of Labour?* London: Tavistock.

—— (1982) The Role of the General Practitioner in Helping the Elderly Widowed. *Journal of the Royal College of General Practitioners* **32**: 215–27.

—— (in press) Prescribing and Communicating. In, J. Hasler and D. Pendleton (eds) *Essays on Doctor-Patient Communication.* London: Academic Press.

CARTWRIGHT, A. and ANDERSON, R. (1981) *General Practice Revisited.* London: Tavistock.

CARTWRIGHT, A. and O'BRIEN, M. (1976) Social Class Variations in Health Care and in the Nature of General Practitioner Consultations. In, Margaret Stacey (ed.) *The Sociology of the NHS.* Sociological Review Monograph 22. University of Keele.

CARTWRIGHT, A., HOCKEY, L., and ANDERSON, J. (1973) *Life before Death.* London: Routledge and Kegan Paul.

CLAYTON, P., DESMARAIS, L., and WINOKUR, G. (1968) A Study of Normal Bereavement. *American Journal of Psychiatry* 125: 168–78.

CUMMING, E. and HENRY, W. E. (1961) *Growing Old: the Process of Disengagement.* New York: Basic Books.

DEPARTMENT OF HEALTH AND SOCIAL SECURITY (1977) *Family Expenditure Survey Analyses.* London: HMSO.

—— (1978) *Drug Master Index* (Straight Alpha). London: HMSO.

—— (1980) *Health and Personal Social Services Statistics for England 1978.* London: HMSO.

DUFF, R. S. and HOLLINGSHEAD, A. B. (1968) *Sickness and Society.* New York: Harper and Row.

DUNNELL, K. and CARTWRIGHT, A. (1972) *Medicine Takers, Prescribers and Hoarders.* London and Boston: Routledge and Kegan Paul.

GENERAL REGISTER OFFICE (1967) *The Registrar General's Statistical Review of England Wales for the Year 1966.* Part 1, Tables Medical. London: HMSO.

GLASER, B. G. and STRAUSS, A. L. (1965) *Awareness of Dying.* London: Weidenfeld and Nicolson.

—— (1968) *Time for Dying.* Chicago, Ill.: Aldine.

GLICK, I. O., WEISS, R. S., and PARKES, C. M. (1974) *The First Year of Bereavement.* New York: John Wiley and Sons.

GORER, G. (1965) *Death, Grief and Mourning.* London: Cresset Press.

GRAY, P. G. and CORLETT, T. (1950) Sampling for the Social survey. *Journal of the Royal Statistical Society, Series A (General)* CXIII(11).

HART, J. T. (1971) The Inverse Care Law. *Lancet* 1: 405–12.

HENDRICKS, J. and HENDRICKS, C. D. (1978) Ageism and Common Stereotypes. In, V. Carver and P. Liddiard (eds) *An Aging Population.* London: Hodder and Stoughton.

HINTON, J. (1967) *Dying.* Harmondsworth: Penguin Books.

—— (1980) Whom Do Dying Patients Tell? *British Medical Journal* 281: 1328–330.

HOLMES, T. H. and RAHE, R. H. (1967) The Social Readjustment Rating Scale. *Journal of Psychosomatic Research* 11 (2): 213–18.

HOOPER, D. and INEICHEN, B. (1979) Adjustment to Moving: A Follow-up Study of the Mental Health of Young Families in New Housing. *Social Science and Medicine* 13D (3): 163–68.

HUNT, A. (1978) *The Elderly at Home. A Study of People Aged Sixty-Five and Over Living in the Community in England in 1976.* London: HMSO.

ILLICH, I. (1974) *Medical Nemesis: the Expropriation of Health.* London: Calder and Boyars.

ISAACS, B. (1971) Geriatric Patients: Do Their Families Care? *British Medical Journal* 4: 282–86.

ISAACS, B., LIVINGSTONE, M., and NEVILLE, Y. (1972) *Survival of the Unfittest: a Study of Geriatric Patients in Glasgow.* London and Boston: Routledge and Kegan Paul.

JONES, J. S. (1981) Telling the Right Patient. *British Medical Journal* 283: 291–92.

KALISH, R. (1976) Death and Dying in a Social Context. In, R. Binstock and E. Sharas (eds) *Handbook of Aging and the Social Sciences.* New York: Van Nostrand Reinhold.

KALISH, R. and REYNOLDS, D. (1976) *Death and Ethnicity: A Psychocultural Study.* Los Angeles, Calif.: University of Southern California Press.

KAY, D. W., ROTH, M. and HOPKINS, B. (1955) Affective Disorders Arising in the Senium. *Journal of Mental Science* 101: 302–16.

KERCKHOFF, A. C. (1966) Family Patterns and Morale in Retirement. In, I. Simpson and J. McKinney (eds) *Social Aspects of Aging.* Durham, North Carolina: Duke University Press.

KLEIN, R. F., DEAN, A., and BOGDONOFF, M. D. (1967) The Impact of Illness on the Spouse. *Journal of Chronic Diseases* 20: 241–48.

KRAUS, A. S. and LILIENFELD, A. M. (1959) Some Epidemiologic Aspects of the High Mortality Rate in the Young Widowed Group. *Journal of Chronic Diseases* 10: 207–17.

KÜBLER-ROSS, E. (1970) *On Death and Dying.* London: Tavistock.

LINDEMANN, E. (1944) The Symptomatology and Management of Acute Grief. *American Journal of Psychiatry* 101: 141–48.

LOPATA, H. (1971) Widows as a Minority Group. *Gerontologist* 11 (1) (Spring Part 2): 67–77.

——— (1973) *Widowhood in an American City.* Cambridge, Mass: Schenkman.

MACMILLAN, D. (1963) Recent Developments in Community Mental Health. *Lancet* 1: 567–71.

MADDISON, D. and VIOLA, A. (1968) The Health of Widows in the Year Following Bereavement. *Journal of Psychosomatic Research* 12: 297–306.

MARRIS, P. (1958) *Widows and Their Families.* London: Routledge and Kegan Paul.

——— (1974) *Loss and Change.* London: Routledge and Kegan Paul.

NOVACK, D. H., PLUMER, R., SMITH, R. L., OCHITILL, H., MORROW, G. R., and BENNETT, J. M. (1979) Changes in Physicians' Attitudes toward Telling the Cancer Patient. *Journal of the American Medical Association* 241: 897–900.

OFFICE OF POPULATION CENSUSES AND SURVEYS (1964) *Census 1961. England and Wales Household Composition Tables.* London: HMSO.

——— (1978a) *Demographic Review: A Report on Population in Great Britain.* London: HMSO.

——— (1978b) *Marriage and Divorce Statistics 1975 for England and Wales.* London: HMSO.

——— (1979) *Mortality Statistics 1977.* London: HMSO.

PARISH, P. (1976) *Medicines. A guide for everybody.* London: Allen Lane.

244 Life After A Death

PARKES, C. M. (1964) Recent Bereavement as a Cause of Mental Illness. *British Journal of Psychiatry* 110: 198–204.

—— (1965) Bereavement and Mental Illness. *British Journal of Medical Psychology* 38: 1–26.

—— (1970) The First Year of Bereavement. A Longitudinal Study of the Reaction of London Widows to the Death of Their Husband. *Psychiatry* 33: 444–67.

—— (1972) *Bereavement*. London: Tavistock.

—— (1979) Evaluation of a Bereavement Service. In, A. De Vries and A. Carni (eds) *The Dying Human*. Ramat Gan, Israel: Turtledove.

—— (1980) Bereavement Counselling: Does it Work? *British Medical Journal* 281: 3–6.

PARKES, C. M., BENJAMIN, B., and FITZGERALD, R. G. (1969) Broken Heart: A Statistical Study of Increased Mortality Among Widowers. *British Medical Journal* 1: 740–43.

PARKES, C. M. and BROWN, R. (1972) Health after Bereavement: A Controlled Study of Young Boston Widows and Widowers. *Psychosomatic Medicine* 34: 449–61.

RAINWATER, L. (1965) *Family Design*. Chicago, Ill.: Aldine Press.

RAPHAEL, B. (1977) Preventive Intervention with the Recently Bereaved. *Archives of General Psychiatry* 34: 1450–454.

REES, W. D. and LUTKINS, S. G. (1967) Mortality of Bereavement. *British Medical Journal* 4: 13–16.

RILEY, M. and FONER, A. (1968) *Aging & Society*. Volume 1. An Inventory of Research Findings. New York: Russell Sage Foundation.

ROBINSON, D. (1981) Personal Communication.

SAUNDERS, C. M. (1966) The Management of Terminal Illness. *Hospital Medicine* 1: 225–28.

SHANAS, E., TOWNSEND, P., WEDDERBURN, D., FRIIS, H., MILHØJ, P., and STEHOUWER, J. (1968) *Old People in Three Industrial Societies*. London: Routledge and Kegan Paul.

STEIN, Z. and SUSSER, M. (1969) Widowhood and Mental Illness. *British Journal of Preventive and Social Medicine* 23: 106–10.

TOWNSEND, P. (1957) *The Family Life of Old People*. London: Routledge and Kegan Paul.

TUNSTALL, J. (1966) *Old and Alone*. London: Routledge and Kegan Paul.

WICKS, M. (1978) *Old and Cold*. London: Heinemann Educational Books.

WILKES, E. (1965) Terminal Cancer at Home. *Lancet* 1: 799–801.

WILLIAMSON, J., STOKOE, I. H., GRAY, S., FISHER, M., SMITH, A., MCGHEE, A., and STEPHENSON, E. (1964) Old People at Home: Their Unreported Needs. *Lancet* 1: 1117–120.

WILLMOTT, P. and YOUNG, M. (1960) *Family and Class in a London Suburb*. London: Routledge and Kegan Paul.

YOUNG, M., BENJAMIN, B., and WALLIS, C. (1963) The Mortality of Widowers. *Lancet* 2: 454–56.

Name index

Subject index

depression — *cont.*
and relationship with general
practitioner, 113;
and general practitioner's assessment
of symptoms, 128–29;
and keeping in touch with friends and
relatives, 188;
and impact on familiars, 195;
see also symptoms
deputizing service, 132–33, 136–39
diet, *see* food
disability among widow(er)s and need
for help, 170;
see also mobility problems and
personal care
district nurse, *see* nurse
diuretics, *see* cardiovascular and diuretic
drugs
dressing:
help needed by deceased, 24;
help needed by widow(er)s, 99, 193
drugs, classification, 239;
see also medicine taking and
prescribing

education, medical, 223–24;
see also training for general practice

familiars:
definition, 10;
composition of sample, 13;
and help in caring for deceased,
40–3;
and views on role of general
practitioner, 117–19;
and views about marital relationship
and adjustment of widower, 143,
161–63;
and help and support for widowed,
190–211;
age and domestic responsibilities, 191
feet, trouble with, 97–100, 131, 158,
193
finance:
financial effects of deceased's illness,
39–40;
financial worries, 71–2, 74, 85, 102,
150–51, 153, 173, 228;
management of income and
expenditure, 85–7;
financial situation after death of
spouse, 88–90;

expense of social activities, 188,
215–17;
financial help for telephone, 218
food, 40, 81, 88;
diet of widow(er), 90–1;
assessment by general practitioners,
130
forgetfulness, 97–100, 104, 128–29;
see also mental confusion and
symptoms
frequency of contact with children,
siblings, and others, 172–75,
182–85, 188;
with general practitioner, *see*
consultations
friends and neighbours:
as familiars, 13;
and help with care of deceased, 24;
discussion about death and illness of
deceased, 50, 59;
and help with meals, 91;
and support for widow(er), 169–82,
184, 188, 192–93, 221;
and need for companionship, 214

gardening, 81–6, 192
general practitioners:
characteristics of sample doctors,
8–10;
care of deceased, 22–3, *25–34*,
122–31;
as informant about death and illness,
49, 52, 56, *57–63*, 134;
care of bereaved, 93–5, 102–09,
111–31, 221–24;
attitudes, *132–40*
geriatric hospital, 30
Gingerbread, organization for single
parent families, 226
grandchildren, 177–79
grief, *see* bereavement, emotional
reactions to
guilt, *see* bereavement, emotional
reactions to

headaches, 97–100, 158;
see also symptoms
health of familiars, 194
health of widow(er), 80, *93*, *96–105*,
203–10, 240;
and restriction on activities while
caring for spouse, 36;
and thoughts of moving house, 76;

For Product Safety Concerns and Information please contact our EU
representative GPSR@taylorandfrancis.com
Taylor & Francis Verlag GmbH, Kaufingerstraße 24, 80331 München, Germany